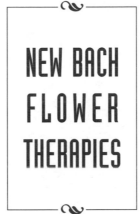

NEW BACH FLOWER THERAPIES

NEW BACH FLOWER THERAPIES

∾

HEALING THE

EMOTIONAL AND

SPIRITUAL CAUSES

OF ILLNESS

∾

DIETMAR KRÄMER

TRANSLATED BY HANS-GEORG BAKKER

HEALING ARTS PRESS
ROCHESTER, VERMONT

Healing Arts Press
One Park Street
Rochester, Vermont 05767
www.gotoit.com

First published in German under the title *Neue Therapien mit Bach-Blüten 1*
by Ansata-Verlag, Interlaken, Switzerland.
Copyright © 1989 by Ansata-Verlag
Translation copyright © 1995 by Healing Arts Press

Note to the reader: This book is intended as an informational guide. The remedies,
approaches, and techniques described herein are meant to supplement, and not to be a
substitute for, professional medical care or treatment. They should not be used to treat a
serious ailment without prior consultation with a qualified health care professional.

LIBRARY OF CONGRESS CATALOGING-IN-PUBLICATION DATA
Krämer, Dietmar.
[Neue Therapien mit Bach-Blüten 1. English]
New Bach flower therapies: healing the emotional and spiritual causes of illness /
Dietmar Krämer; translated by Hans-Georg Bakker.
p. cm.
Translation of: Neue Therapien mit Bach-Blüten 1.
Includes bibliographical references and index.
ISBN 0-89281-529-9
1. Flowers—Therapeutic use.
2. Bach, Edward, 1886–1936. I. Title
RX615.F55K7313   1995
615'.321–dc20   94–49148
CIP

Printed and bound in the United States

10 9 8 7 6 5 4 3 2

This book was typeset in Optima with Industria as the display typeface

Healing Arts Press is a division of Inner Traditions International

Distributed to the book trade in Canada by Publishers Group West (PGW),
Toronto, Ontario
Distributed to the book trade in the United Kingdom by Deep Books, London
Distributed to the book trade in Australia by Millennium Books, Newtown, N.S.W.
Distributed to the book trade in New Zealand by Tandem Press, Auckland
Distributed to the book trade in South Africa by Alternative Books, Ferndale

CONTENTS

PREFACE

With the publication of Dr. Edward Bach's *Heal Thyself* in 1931, a new era in the history of medicine began. Yet Edward Bach was to endure the fate of many other pioneers of genius: his healing method remained almost unknown for the next decades, despite the great accomplishments he and his successors were able to make.

It was not until forty-eight years later that his books *Heal Thyself* and *The Twelve Healers,* along with Dr. F. J. Wheeler's *The Bach Remedies Repertory,* were published in German translation. In the last two years eight new books and three new editions have been published in German on the subject.

The present book is titled *New Bach Flower Therapies.* Why "new" therapies? The answer is simple: new therapeutic consequences—the result of practical work with the patient and a sensitive approach—have opened up entirely new possibilities for Bach Flower Therapy in both diagnosis and application. A new treatment method, based on the ideas of the "tracks" and Bach Flower skin zones, has also developed into an independent therapy.

This new therapeutic concept is based on four principal elements, as described below.

CONSIDERATION OF THE RELATIONSHIP AMONG THE FLOWERS
ॐ

Through the relationship of the flowers to each other (the "tracks") it is possible to determine which flower covers the superficial side of a problem and which focuses more on the deeper cause. In this way a new hierarchy is created, one that will determine the therapy to follow. This hierarchy is especially helpful when a patient needs many flowers, which can make it difficult to find a starting point. Once the acute problems have diminished, it is possible with the help of this hierarchy to determine which of the deeper negative emotional states have led to the present complaints. It is then possible, if desired, to continue the therapy with the appropriate flowers to open up the mind.

ASTROLOGICAL DIAGNOSIS

Astrological psychology offers the opportunity to recognize deeper-lying emotional conflicts unknown to the patient. Thus it offers valuable diagnostic help, especially for children, who are unable to recount a case history. The astrological diagnosis often provides the essential clue to the emotional reason for an illness.

Peter Damian, in his book *The Twelve Healers of the Zodiac: The Astrology Handbook of the Bach Flower Therapies,* describes the use of twelve of the thirty-eight Bach Flowers in astrological diagnosis. With the new concept of "tracks" it is possible to incorporate thirty-two of the flowers. Five of the remaining six flowers deal with external causes and influences and therefore are easy to recognize.

DIAGNOSIS THROUGH THE BACH FLOWER BODY MAPS

Every Bach Flower Remedy is related to an area on the surface of the body— similar to the foot reflex zones. Negative moods lead to a change of energetic structure in these places, which often is accompanied by pain and disturbing sensations. Thus, solely by pinpointing the areas on the body map it is possible to obtain a flower diagnosis.

APPLICATION OF THE FLOWERS TO THE SKIN

Through a direct application to the disturbed areas it is possible to increase the effect of the flowers tremendously. Not only is it possible to improve negative emotional states much faster in this way than through oral tinctures, but the physical complaints often ease immediately as well. Bach Flower Therapy is thus not only a soul cleanser "to harmonize the psyche," as is often stated, but also a therapy for the treatment of physical ailments.

New Bach Flower Therapies explores the interrelationships among the flowers and describes the astrological diagnosis, relating both to the already known application of flowers. A subsequent volume will be dedicated to the Bach Flower body maps. The descriptions of the flowers incorporate original quotations from patients to create a more lively image of the flowers.

1

The Bach Flower Remedies

Edward Bach (1886–1936) was a British physician and well-known pathologist, immunologist, and bacteriologist. His discoveries in these areas of medicine were pioneering, and his innovative bacterial vaccines have found a permanent place in homeopathic medicine under the name "Bach nosodes." Despite his medical successes, he still felt unsatisfied. For him an illness was not just a "dysfunction of the human machine" but an effect of disharmony between body and mind. The symptoms of an illness were the external expression, the bodily manifestation, of negative emotional states.

His postulate was, "Treat the person, not the illness." He assumed that the causes of disease were negative emotional states such as sorrow, fear, dissatisfaction, impatience, sadness, and so forth. Therefore, he started looking for soul remedies that could influence the causes of an illness.

A great nature lover, Edward Bach was also extremely sensitive. In his quest for new remedies he would go into the countryside, pick the petal of a single flower, and lay it on his tongue. With the help of his immense sensitivity he was able to feel the effect of a plant on the human body and psyche. In this way he found the plants he thought were useful for the treatment of negative emotional states. He used not only the blossoms of wildflowers but also the flowers of wild shrubs, bushes, and trees.

The production of his remedies is handled in two ways: Using the "sun method," the flowers are picked on a warm summer day in full sunshine. The flowers are put in a glass bowl with fresh spring water, taken, if possible, from a spring close to the location of the flower. It is sufficient that the flowers only cover the surface of the water. The bowl is placed in the sun for two to four hours. According to Edward Bach the sun will transfer the vibration of the flowers into the medium of the water, which in this way becomes energetically impregnated.

Afterward the flowers are removed from the solution, and an equal portion of alcohol is added for preservation (Bach used brandy). The derived solution is stored in a stock bottle. During treatment, the remedy is usually diluted with water.

Since not all flowers, shrubs, bushes, and trees bloom at a time of year with plenty of sunshine, a second method for the preparation of remedies is necessary, the so-called cooking method. The flowers and buds are picked according to the sun method and boiled down. The extract is filtered several times and mixed again with the same portion of alcohol as a preservative. The process is continued in the same way as the remedies produced with the sun method.

According to Edward Bach, illness is "solely and purely corrective; it is neither vindictive nor cruel, but is the means adopted by our own Souls to point out to us our faults, to prevent our making greater errors, to hinder us from doing more harm, and to bring us back to that path of Truth and Light from which we should never have strayed."[1]

At a different place he writes: "If you suffer from stiffness of joint or limb, you can be equally certain that there is stiffness in your mind; that you are rigidly holding on to some idea, some principle, some convention maybe, which you should not have. If you suffer from asthma, or difficulty in breathing, you are in some way stifling another personality; or from lack of courage to do right, smothering yourself."[2]

And again: "Even the part of the body affected indicates the nature of the fault. The hand, failure or wrong in action; the foot, failure to assist others; the brain, lack of control; the heart, deficiency or excess or wrong doing in the aspect of love; the eye, failure to see aright and comprehend the truth when placed before you."[3] This observation evokes the so-called language of the body, well known to us all in sayings such as the following:

- ❧ Chills going up one's spine
- ❧ Butterflies in one's stomach
- ❧ Being heartbroken
- ❧ Something hard to swallow
- ❧ The load on one's shoulders

Edward Bach assumed that thirty-eight "virtues" serve as links between the personality and the higher self. The expression "the higher self" is well known in the esoteric teachings of every culture and every religion. It represents our higher authority. Suffering, according to these teachings, originates when a person is not in tune with his or her higher self, a state that, according to Bach, will change virtues into negative images. This process, for example, will turn:

- ∾ Courage and faith into fears
- ∾ Self-esteem into inferiority complexes
- ∾ Cheerfulness into melancholy
- ∾ Humility into arrogance
- ∾ Forgiveness into blame
- ∾ Hope into hopelessness and despair
- ∾ Belief into disbelief and pessimism

Bach Flowers reestablish one's contact with the higher self through their vibrations and help one to regain his or her lost virtue. These negative emotional states are not "fought" as symptoms, because that would maintain them energetically. Instead, they are inundated by superior harmonic vibrations of energy that, according to Edward Bach, melt them away like "snow in the sunshine."[4]

The thirty-eight Bach Flowers belong to the "flowers of higher rank," as he called them. Each of them embodies a certain concept of mind and like a sort of catalyst restores the blocked contact between the soul and the personality.[5]

The forthcoming *New Bach Flower Body Maps* focuses on the theory of negative emotional states and their effects on the physiology of the human body. Edward Bach divided these negative emotional states into seven groups:

1. Fear
2. Insecurity
3. Lack of interest in the present
4. Loneliness
5. Vulnerability to ideas and influences
6. Despondency and despair
7. Excessive concern for the well-being of others

A different classification of the flowers, which in my experience is more suited for practical use, is described in this book.

2

A New Classification of the Flowers

Bach Flowers can be divided into two groups: the inner and outer flowers.

Outer Flowers
∾

The outer flowers treat negative emotional states that develop as a result of or are a reaction to external influences. They include:

1. Results of emotional shock, injury, or disappointment
2. Fear of being unable to meet an external challenge (driving test, final exams, daily work demands, etc.)
3. Feelings of insecurity or uncertainty owing to a new phase in one's life, such as puberty, menopause, new career, move, marriage, divorce, unexpected pregnancy, or climate change
4. Despair in a seemingly hopeless situation
5. Vague, abstract fears resulting from astral or celestial influences, which are perceived as threats because they are incomprehensible

The recognition of these negative emotional states is very important, because they are readily apparent and therefore must be treated first. Treatment of deeper emotional problems is possible only if external influences can be taken on and processed again normally. Continuous confrontation with the surrounding environment will otherwise hinder the resolution of deeper-lying emotional conflicts.

INNER FLOWERS

ᙇ

The inner flowers can be divided into twelve groups, or "tracks." Within each track is one communication flower, one compensation flower, and one decompensation flower. All twelve tracks have one base flower in common. This flower cannot be categorized and is used solely by indication.

Communication Flowers

The communication flowers correspond with our individual characters. They represent the way we communicate with our environment.

If we act in harmony with our higher self, the flowers embody positive emotional concepts such as courage, kindness, humility, and so forth. If the communication with our higher self is blocked, however, our communication with our environment is disturbed and we react with insecurity, fear, impatience, arrogance, and so on. Thus we live the negative emotional state of these flowers, which leads to further problems. Yet there are no problems per se, only situations. A situation becomes a problem only when we can no longer handle it. Negative emotional states offer a chance to recognize and transform them and in this way reestablish our connection with the higher self.

Compensation Flowers

If the lesson of the communication flowers is not learned, we try to compensate for this fault. Insecurity, for example, represented by the negative concept of the Cerato flower, is compensated either with confidence and the demonstration of strength or the need for power, dominance, and, in extreme cases, tyranny. Such an artificial state of mind cannot be maintained for long. In this example the person will regress from her deceptive strength to a state of total insecurity and aimlessness, as embodied by the Wild Oat flower.

Decompensation Flowers

States of decompensation are psychopathological end states. Those in such a state experience it as a dark hole into which they have fallen and out of which they cannot climb with their own strength. The recognition and treatment of these emotional states, in conjunction with the external flower remedies, has absolute priority. The states of decompensation are obstructions that can be found not only in Bach Flower Therapy but also in other forms of therapy, such as acupuncture, homeopathy, and psychotherapy.

Wild Rose patients, for example, will rarely respond to therapy, because they are rooted in a condition of capitulation, inner abdication, and resignation. This emotional state affects the whole body, especially the circulation. These people suffer from extremely low blood pressure that cannot be stimulated even by strong coffee or appropriate medications. The accompanying fatigue also cannot be eliminated by plenty of sleep, fresh air, cold packs, or other methods. After taking Wild Rose, many of these patients report an instantaneous feeling of wakefulness and clarity. Sometimes they refer to the image of a light bulb being switched on.

Other states of decompensation are:

- Deep despair
- Feelings of guilt
- Extreme insecurity and aimlessness
- Longing for the past as an escape from reality
- Periods of deep despondency and melancholy, without apparent reason
- Extreme physical and psychological tension
- The feeling of going crazy combined with compulsive acts
- The feeling of being innerly impure and unclean
- Tormenting thoughts that continuously repeat themselves and cannot be shut off and pushed aside
- Censorship, arrogance, and intolerance

The elimination of these decompensatory states is therefore the primary therapeutic goal. Only then is it possible for the mind to work on deeper layers of consciousness.

Although it is possible to alleviate deeper negative emotional states such as lack of willpower, insecurity, and impatience without the use of decompensation flowers therapy remains incomplete and success is only modest. In most cases the negative states of decompensation are described by the patient as the most urgent problems and therefore cannot be overlooked.

In the following chapters the twelve groups of inner flowers are presented in detail. I have named them "tracks" because emotional problems run as if on a railroad track, from a state of communication to a state of compensation and then to a state of decompensation.

3

INNER FLOWERS: THE TWELVE TRACKS

CENTAURY—HOLLY—PINE

Centaury *(Centaurium umbellatum)*

Centaury people are charming and considerate, loved everywhere for their kindness and helpfulness. The motivation behind their "noble" character traits is the desire for appreciation and love. Out of fear of hurting someone and thereby losing appreciation and love, they show so much consideration that they often lose their own will. Self-determination and self-fulfillment are sacrificed for appreciation and devotion. They value helpfulness and service to others at the expense of their own interests. The loss of appreciation and love strikes so much terror in them that they ultimately become willing slaves of a dominant personality.

These people often describe themselves in the followings ways:

- ∾ I am good natured.
- ∾ I don't want to hurt anybody.
- ∾ My will is not very strong.
- ∾ I often find it difficult to say no.
- ∾ I am easily talked into something and get angry about it afterward.
- ∾ I often don't find the right moment in a relationship to say, "Enough, no more!"

- ❧ I have always lived for others and have denied my own needs.
- ❧ I never have the courage to disagree.
- ❧ I grew up late.
- ❧ I am afraid of not fulfilling another person's expectations, even when the other person has not expressed her expectations.
- ❧ I often feel that I have been used.
- ❧ When I want something it is hard for me to express it.
- ❧ I am cowardly and am tyrannized by others.
- ❧ I often ask myself, "Why don't you fight back?"
- ❧ I often say yes because I am afraid of no longer being loved if I express my opinion.
- ❧ I need recognition.
- ❧ I am afraid of being rejected.
- ❧ I am afraid to assert myself.
- ❧ I am afraid of being repelled.

People who live in a Centaury state often have a weak handshake.

Fundamentally, Centaury has to do with demarcation, on a personal as well as energetic level. On the personal level it is the demarcation of one's own will from the will of another. If she is not successful, the individual will become an instrument of another stronger personality because of her lack of willpower. On the energetic level it is the demarcation of one's energy field from its surroundings. If demarcation is not attained, the individual will suffer apparently unexplainable fatigue. She will, for example, report feeling tired and weak in front of other people. The fear that other people can drain one's energy is sometimes expressed. Centaury can be a great help here, by closing the aura and protecting the energy body and the personality from the influences of the immediate surroundings. Anyone who feels tired and drained in the presence of others is advised to squeeze one pure drop of Centaury directly from the stock bottle onto the tongue. One will immediately feel awake again and recharged with energy. Centaury in conjunction with Walnut is also a proven remedy that protects one from the influences of the so-called astral sphere.

A small bottle of Centaury should be present in every treatment room. Even strong-willed therapists can fall into a Centaury state, for example, by feeling too much empathy for their unfortunate patients. Very ill patients will automatically drain energy from their surroundings, as a result of the energy imbalance caused by their extreme weakness. A therapist who is exhausted by one patient will not be much help for other patients. Fortunately, this can be stopped by a few drops of Centaury.

To sacrifice oneself in this way for other people is not worthwhile. We can help only from a position of strength. Götz Blome writes on this issue: "Every sacrifice that is made out of weakness, that does not originate from conviction and one's inner law (and is therefore no sacrifice) is not only worthless but also harmful. Through its inner falsehood it will ruin both the giving and receiving person."[1]

To repeat the basic idea of the Centaury flower once more: In a Centaury state, patients show little resistance to either a material or the ethereal environment. Centaury closes up and anchors the aura on a subtle level. On the level of the personality it results in stabilization. Therefore, Centaury is one of the most important Bach Flowers. In the truest sense of the word, it helps one lead an independent life.

Holly *(Ilex aquifolium)*

The flower remedy Holly helps against anger, hate, envy, jealousy, suspicion, and revengefulness.

Holly people live in a constant state of restless irritation, get angry easily, and often lose control of themselves. Even a fly on the wall will anger them in situations of extreme tension. They often complain about others, whom they blame for their own bad mood. Generally, they always find a culprit whom they can blame for their own mistakes.

Holly people report about themselves:

- ∾ I easily fly into a rage. Sometimes I am so tense that even a small thing makes me mad.
- ∾ I often get angry at myself, especially when someone has persuaded me to do something I actually do not want to do.
- ∾ I often have uncontrollable temper tantrums.
- ∾ I am constantly unsatisfied and suffer for no reason.
- ∾ My friends say I am hot-tempered.
- ∾ Sometimes I am very unfriendly, although the other person has given me no reason to be.
- ∾ I often wake up at night to my own voice and hear myself complaining out loud.
- ∾ I am very resentful.
- ∾ It is difficult for me to forgive myself or others.
- ∾ I am very suspicious.
- ∾ I am very jealous. When my husband went to a seminar, he had to call home every hour.
- ∾ I often envy other women who are prettier than I am.

As a result of their temperament, Holly people often suffer acute and violent illnesses—for example, sudden high fevers; inflamed, burning, or itching skin rashes; allergies; and gallblader disease. Coughing (Do not breathe on me) and vomiting (This is making me sick) are acts of aggression and expressions of a Holly state of mind.

How do these extremely destructive states of mind originate? It is said that hate is the mirror image of love. Why does a person shut herself off from love? Is she afraid of love? Does she want to protect herself? Did she once show too much emotion toward other people and was so disappointed by others—and possibly also by herself—that she is afraid of her feelings? Is that what Holly people try to express when they say, "I cannot easily forgive myself or others"?

Let us remember the image of Centaury. These people offer so much empathy to their environment that often they cannot say no. They give a lot, live almost solely for others but expect to receive the feeling of acknowledgment and being loved from them. If these people are disappointed—they also often describe the feeling of being used—they have two possibilities: Either they learn life's lessons by exercising their own will and taking their lives into their own hands, or they compensate for their weakness by blocking out the emotions by which they were hurt. Devotion turns into resentment. Necessary demarcation from the world turns into separation. Because one's own will is weak, it has to be defended constantly from other people. We attack other people, however, only when we believe they will impede us in some way.

The mistake these people make is that they ward off love and affection. They reject the one thing they need most. In the Centaury state they long so much for love and acknowledgment that they will do anything for other people, just to receive this feeling. They even repress their own needs out of fear of not being able to fulfill the needs of the other person and thus losing the other's love and affection.

The first step is to free the blocked feelings with the Holly flower. One should not stop on this level, however, because the cause lies deeper. Only by treating Centaury's negative emotional stage can the real basis for the destructive feelings of the Holly state be eliminated. Altogether, Holly is the compensation remedy for the comunication flower Centaury. Centaury represents, in Chinese terms, an extreme yin state. An imbalance is always unstable and cannot exist on its own for long; therefore a compensation will eventually occur, which means that the equilibrium will tip from the extreme yin state into the yang state. This works like the pendulum of a clock, which swings from one side to the other and back again.

Since the yin in the Centaury state was extreme, the compensatory yang in the Holly state is just as extreme. The patient accordingly overreacts. If this state is not overcome it will tilt back from the extreme yang to the extreme yin. What follows is the state of decompensation, the Pine state.

Pine *(Pinus sylvestris)*

People who need the pine flower constantly suffer from a guilty conscience. In every possible and impossible life situation, they find reasons to feel guilty. Even when successful they accuse themselves of not being good enough. If they get criticized they torture themselves with self-accusations. When they are praised, they cannot accept the praise. Often they say:

- That isn't worth mentioning.
- That was nothing special.
- After all, it was my duty.

They have a hard time accepting presents, because they believe that they do not deserve them. Their phrases often begin with:

- If only I had . . .
- Why did I . . .
- Please excuse me for . . .
- I am very sorry that . . .

Pine people say about themselves:

- I often have a guilty conscience.
- I look for faults in myself, even when it actually might have been someone else's fault.
- In unpleasant situations I always convince myself that I am to blame.
- I often remember unpleasant situations from the past and still feel guilty today. Sometimes it gets so bad that I could jump out of my own skin. I feel it physically and start to tense up throughout my body.
- I still suffer from the bad lifestyle I used to have.
- I often blame myself now for eveything I did not do for my children.
- I often blame myself for not giving my children enough love.
- I often accuse myself.
- I criticize myself when I can't perform.
- Even when I am sick, I have a guilty concience. If the medication does not work, I immediately think that it is my own fault.
- It is sometimes difficult for me to be really happy because I am always conscious of what I have missed out on.
- I have many guilty feelings about sex.

∾ I often blame myself for other people's mistakes.

∾ If other people do not say much, I accuse myself of insulting or hurting them. Even when they deny it I still feel guilty, because I imagine that they will not admit it out of courtesy and consideration.

∾ I can't be really happy about something and thus often feel sad and depressed. When others call me a party pooper, I feel guilty again.

∾ Often I can't fall asleep because I am tortured by self-accusations. When I am dead tired and not able to function the next morning, I really feel guilty.

∾ If I refuse to do someone a favor, I later have a guilty conscience.

The Pine image contains strong masochistic elements. The patient thinks he must constantly punish himself. What causes such a self-destructive misconception? Let us remember that Pine is the state that follows Holly. In the Holly state the individual always tries to blame someone else. Holly people are never satisfied with other people, which causes them to be constantly tense and aggressive. Pine people are never satisfied with themselves and focus their aggression on themselves.

Pine is the decompensation state of the Centaury flower. In the Centaury state it is difficult for individuals to say no. In the Holly state they fall into the other extreme and always say no, in return for which they will feel guilty in the Pine state.

At first there is a search for love and approval. This desire often leads to a complete loss of self. Eventually, it leads to a point where these individuals feel used by others and start to separate themselves in an aggressive way. Through this demarcation, however, love and approval will be taken away from them. Therefore it is impossible to sustain the Holly state over a long period. They fall back into decompensation and guilty feelings. For many people this becomes a vicious circle; they do not dare say no because of their feelings of guilt. They are taken advantage of again, and the whole game starts over.

Feelings of guilt are the result of a preceding Centaury state. They are always preceded by an act of weakness, in which someone else's blame is taken. A popular saying in such a case is, Why did you let this happen to you?

For the treatment of Centaury states it must first be determined whether the individuals are already in the decompensation phase. Otherwise the will-power gained through the application of Centaury could lead to the reinforcement of guilt. They get scared and complain that the treatment had changed them in a "negative" way, which is then confirmed by their environment.

At first it seems to be a "negative" change when a person who always has put up with everything suddenly rebels and shows his own will. People around him are not always aware that this person was in fact being exploited.

It is important to support the person in these necessary changes and through conversation to help him explain his change of mind.

Decompensation flower	Pine
Compensation flower	Holly
Communication flower	Centaury

CERATO—VINE—WILD OAT

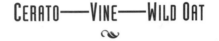

Cerato (*Ceratostigma willmottian*)

Cerato people are curious and industrious. In their enthusiasm they read many books and attend continuing education courses. In school, in seminars, or in lectures they ask a lot of questions, which in certain cases can be stimulating for the lecturer. Many times the questions will be so detailed that one wonders what use the person can get from this information. Sometimes one has the feeling that questions are asked just for the sake of asking.

At the doctor's or the practitioner's they often want to know the diagnosis and the exact laboratory results and sometimes write them down. Sometimes they even have checklists on which they cross out every question, so they will not forget anything. Many times they also have questions about the treatment method, its effects, risks, and successes. Often they want to see examples of successfully treated patients. Sometimes they want to have an extra appointment just to clear up the questions. They often seek the advice of many therapists simultaneously, and they often get confused because of the different opinions they hear. Eventually they read the specialized literature or even attend medical lectures to obtain clarity.

A large part of the suffering of a Cerato person does not originate from physical ailments but from the uncertainty of their illness. If they are attracted to occult teachings, they may start to use divination for every decision. This may even lead to a downright dependency on the radiaesthetic instrument, which is misinterpreted as "inspiration." In this way the addiction to information expands into invisible areas.

What are the reasons behind this excessive hunger for information? Basically, this shows an extremely strong insecurity, especially in the ability to make judgments and decisions. Because the affected persons do not trust their opinions, they ask others for advice. It is exactly this insecurity, however, that makes life so difficult for them. Despite their own knowledge, they are easily misled by others, because they believe that others know better.

Cerato people describe themselves as follows:

- ∾ I often need a lot of time for my decisions and ask other people for advice.
- ∾ The opinion of others is of great importance to me.
- ∾ I often doubt my own decisions.
- ∾ I need external support when I want to act on my decision.
- ∾ I feel insecure if someone opposes my opinion.
- ∾ I am often influenced by other people's opinions.
- ∾ I am very dependent.
- ∾ I am often undecided in my opinions.
- ∾ I spend most of my free time reading.

What is the cause of this inner insecurity and lack of independence, which lead to a more or less conscious dependency on others? It is the refusal of the personality to accept impulses from the inner self. Instead it looks for the truth in the outer world. To a certain extent inspiration and intuition are consciously pushed aside. In the long run, however, nothing is completely lost in our consciousness. Everything we try to push aside pushes back at us, especially in the mirror, through which we constantly face our surroundings.

By noticing the reaction of their family and friends, Cerato individuals recognize how they make fools out of themselves with their constant questioning. It is also not a secret that this is a nuisance to other people. Just the fact that they will experience rejection instead of affection in the long run will force them to find a solution for their problem. Two possibilities exist in this regard: on the one hand, they may accept the chance to learn, listen to their inner voice, start making decisions, and be willing to take responsibility for them. This also includes the willingness to make mistakes and to stick with it. On the other hand, they may be forced to disguise their insecurity. Through self-confidence and the appearance of strength they may try to compensate for their inner weakness.

Vine *(Vitis vinifera)*

Vine people appear capable and confident. They seem to be natural leaders and to be completely convinced of this themselves. In crisis situations they maintain an overview and save the day with their perceptiveness and presence of mind.

Their strong determination and willpower, however, raise the danger of abusing their abilities for selfish reasons. They usually do not understand accusations of being power hungry and dominant. Because of their "greater abilities" they are convinced that to serve others best they must show them what to do.

Vine people say about themselves:

> ∾ What I demand of others is only in their best interest.
> ∾ I will not give in, even when others refuse.
> ∾ The ends justify the means.
> ∾ I would like to see anyone do better.
> ∾ I am accused of insisting on my rights like a tyrant.

To the outside they present themselves as:

> ∾ strict
> ∾ confident
> ∾ dominant
> ∾ inconsiderate
> ∾ unscrupulous
> ∾ unyielding
> ∾ unable to be in a subordinate position
> ∾ merciless

How is it possible to explain such an inconsiderate state, which under certain circumstances can make other people's lives miserable? We have seen how the insecurity of the Cerato state can be concealed by self-confidence. From a yin state, in which the responsibility for one's own life is given to others, a yang state develops in which people believe they have to take responsibility for others.

Although they asked for other people's opinion in the Cerato state, in the Vine state they now tell others what to do. Whereas before they believed that others are always right, now they insist on their own rights. And while earlier they always followed someone else's authority, now they are convinced of their own authority. Their willpower was already strong in the Cerato state. It was blocked, however, by the misconception that they could find the answers to life's questions and problems in the outer world rather than in their own inner self.

Vine people never admit to their previous state of weakness and insecurity. Their exaggerated behavior is influenced by the fear of leaving themselves vulnerable. A popular idiom is the statement: Showing off is a sign of insecurity. It is possible, however, that the individual is not aware of this state because it is too far in the past—possibly in childhood—or because it was a very short episode.

It also does not matter that the individual believes the Cerato symptoms are not applicable to him, either now or in the past. Sometime in the course of therapy these symptoms will reappear on a conscious level. If one listens very carefully, one can find hidden clues about the Cerato state: for example, the exaggerated eagerness for knowledge, the reading of many books, or the great importance attached to other people's opinions. Although he pretends that he is not really influenced by them, he nevertheless wants to hear them.

As frightening as the extreme Vine state can be for others—especially when one thinks of historical representatives of this state such as Napoleon and Hitler—the state of decompensation can be as devastating for these affected individuals. Previous insecurity that was covered up by self-confidence will now come to a state of extreme disorientation.

Wild Oat *(Bromus ramosus)*

Wild oat people are always on a quest. In their desire to achieve something exceptional they have tried many things but have not yet found the right one. They are unsatisfied with life because they do not have a clearly defined goal before them.

These people often change their jobs, partners, and apartments and start many things without finishing them because they cannot find satisfaction anywhere. Life is monotonous, without peaks, because they cannot find meaning in everything they do. This creates the feeling that life is passing them by and they are wasting their valuable time. They feel unhappy about this situation but do not know how to change it.

Wild Oat people say about themselves:

- ❧ I always have the feeling of emptiness inside, and I'm constantly looking for inner fulfillment.
- ❧ Nothing is fun for me because I don't know what I really want.
- ❧ I don't have any goals in life.
- ❧ I can't find meaning in what I'm doing right now.
- ❧ I'm unhappy because I have the wrong career. I would like to do something different, but I don't know what.
- ❧ I feel unsatisfied because I can't find a goal in my life.
- ❧ Everything is gloomy.
- ❧ I'm waiting for something that never comes.
- ❧ I can't be truly happy because everything that happens around me is ordinary.

This unsuccessful quest for meaning and a goal is often compensated for in self-indulgence (fancy cars, fashion, travel, fine dining) or a career. Afterward these people realize that this also was not the great fulfillment. The feeling of emptiness is dominant; it apparently cannot be filled by anything.

Wild Oat state also finds its expression in physical symptoms, for example:

- ∽ Unspecified symptoms that do not relate to any particular illness
- ∽ Unspecified malaise
- ∽ The feeling of being ill without any concrete symptoms
- ∽ Infections that stop in the beginning phase

The Wild Oat state is characterized by the quest and the wait for one's own call. Although these people believed in the previous Vine state that they were chosen to lead the way, they now fall back on themselves in the Wild Oat state—into a state without goals and orientation. The talent is still as present as in the Vine state but not accessible. Focus and determination are missing.

In summary it can be said: At the beginning is the insecurity of the Cerato state, in which the advice of others is constantly sought. This state is compensated for in the Vine state by the pretense of self-confidence and strength. The end state of this insecurity track is total disorientation, in which even the daily pleasures do not make sense anymore.

Wild Oat is used by many practitioners for clarification when many flowers are used and the affected person does not show any clear tendency.

Decompensation flower	Wild Oat
Compensation flower	Vine
Communication flower	Cerato

SCLERANTHUS—ROCK WATER—CRAB APPLE

∽

Scleranthus *(Scleranthus annuus)*

Scleranthus types are versatile, intellectually stimulating people who can recognize, because of their inner mobility, two sides to an issue. Their flexibility, however, can become their doom when they have to decide between two options. As they always can see both sides of a problem, they have to wrestle with a decision.

After coming to a decision, their mental discussion is still far from over, and thus they run into internal conflict. Often decisions already made will later be reversed. For this reason they appear to be unreliable.

Scleranthus people say about themselves:

- I have difficulty deciding between two alternatives. Sometimes I say that one thing is right, and the next day I say the opposite. Other people accuse me of being unreliable.
- I am extremely moody.
- My mood swings widely—sometimes I'm very euphoric, at other times deeply depressed.
- Every low is followed by a high. I feel then I could embrace the whole world.
- I am often neurotic, almost manic.
- I live in extremes, which demands a lot of energy.
- My physical complaints vary, as does my psyche. Sometimes it hurts here, sometimes there.
- Sometimes I start a job but interrupt it shortly thereafter, only to start something new. Then I feel torn over which of the jobs I should finish first.
- When I leave the house, I often return to check if I turned off the stove. Although I never left the stove on, the doubts always torment me. Several times I drove all the way home, which made me late for work.
- When I park my car I walk around it again to check whether all the doors are locked. After walking away a few steps I turn around to check the doors again just in case I've overlooked an open door. I know that this is nonsense, but I can't change it. My doubts torment me; it is almost like an obsession.
- I walk back and forth restlessly in my apartment; I want to run a lot of errands but I don't know where to start. I would prefer to do everything at once. Because this isn't possible, though, it's very hard for me to decide. As soon as I start one project, I become painfully certain that something else is more important. In this way I'm constantly under pressure and drive myself crazy.
- I often have the feeling that I have missed out on something in my life.

Scleranthus people constantly live with the feeling of sitting on the fence, similar to Goethe's Mephisto, who laments, "There are two souls in my chest," or Shakespeare's *Hamlet*: "To Be or not to be, that is the question."

The inner turmoil and restlessness of these people manifest themselves in nervous and absentminded gestures. In a conversation they often cannot concentrate because they have so many things going through their minds simultaneously. As a result, physical symptoms develop that reflect the unstable state of the psyche:

- ∾ A shift from ravenous hunger to lack of appetite
- ∾ Alternation of diarrhea and constipation
- ∾ Change between overexcitement and extreme fatigue
- ∾ A constant change of symptoms that appear without reason and disappear just as suddenly
- ∾ Pain that moves throughout the body
- ∾ Daytime fatigue and nocturnal insomnia caused by a lack of balance between tension and relaxation
- ∾ Change in blood pressure (sometimes too high, sometimes too low)
- ∾ Disturbances in balance
- ∾ Carsickness, seasickness
- ∾ Vomiting during pregnancy

We already have learned about two other "insecurity" flowers, Cerato and Wild Oat. The best way to explain the difference between these flowers is through an example: Imagine that three different people go into a shoe store. The first one, Wild Oat, stands in front of the shelf and is completely overwhelmed by the great variety. It is even hard for him to pick out a few pairs of shoes for closer selection.

The second one, Cerato, brought someone along to help him with his search. He decisively approaches the shelf and quickly finds the right pair for himself. Now he asks the other person whether these shoes would suit him. If the other person agrees, he buys the shoes at once. If the other disagrees, he is absolutely shaken and may put the shoes back on the shelf. Only when he finds a pair that the other person is convinced will suit him will he buy them. If a Cerato person comes into a store by himself, he seeks confirmation from the salesperson.

The third one, Scleranthus, has found two pairs of shoes from the big assortment of those he likes. To decide on one, however, becomes a big problem. He tries on one pair and is convinced that these are the right ones for him. Just to make sure, however, he also tries on the second pair, and now he leans more toward them. To be really certain he tries on the first pair again, and the whole game starts over. He is completely torn, but in contrast to Cerato he will not ask anyone for help. Instead he struggles with his decision alone.

The symbol for the Scleranthus flower is the scale. Sometimes one side is up, sometimes the other. Because these continuous fluctuations and insecurities turn into a serious problem for the affected person, the pressure of suffering calls for a solution in time. The person starts to look for something that will make the decision for him. This leads to the state of compensation.

Rock Water

Rock water types are people with ideals. They recognize certain things in their lives as being right and try to live according to them. As a result they are very strict with themselves and deny themselves many things that are not consistent with their principles. In their efforts to convince others of their ideals, they often try to be role models.

Rock Water people say about themselves:

    ∾ I have high expectations and therefore often have to make sacrifices.
    ∾ I have extremely moral ideas.
    ∾ My notions of morality often do not coincide with my desires. Therefore, I often have to suppress them.
    ∾ I wish that other people would appreciate what I do.
    ∾ I want to live according to my ideals.
    ∾ I try to do everything perfectly, to be an example for others.
    ∾ I want to be seen by others as good.

Rock Water people focus on their principles, on "doing the right thing." Their idealism often tends toward fanaticism and their need to convince others of their "message" is often expressed in their membership in extremist groups or sects.

Representatives are, for example:

    ∾ Strict vegetarians who, when invited to dinner, eat only potatoes and salad to be faithful to their principles
    ∾ Strict macrobiotics who bring their own meals to friends, so as not to be tempted to go against their principles
    ∾ Strict teetotalers, who do not even drink a sip of wine at Holy Communion
    ∾ Strict antismokers, who continuously avoid secondhand smoke and even refuse invitations to places where people smoke
    ∾ Religious extremists who want to become holy while still on earth
    ∾ Candidates for enlightenment who devote all their time to yoga and meditation exercises and completely give up

worldly pleasures such as socializing, bowling, and going to the movies or the theater

∾ Homeopaths who spend hours looking through books for "the one remedy" and who prescribe a single remedy on a trial basis when the symptoms are unclear, rather than give the patient a mixture for fast relief

It is hard for these people to recognize that these firm preconceptions make their lives not easier but more complicated. In their attempt to end the insecurity and doubts of the Scleranthus state by coming to a definite decision, they have robbed themselves of the opportunity to act according to their own free will. Instead of freeing themselves from the "agony of choice," they become slaves of their own ironclad decisions. Out of fear of losing control and falling back into the unstable Scleranthus state, they are not able to give up their ideals.

In time this rigid holding on to principles also expresses itself in physical embodiments of disease such as stiffness of the joints and arteriosclerosis. Even Paracelsus had the opinion that rigid thoughts lead to stiff joints. The continuous suppression of the libido leads in time to a total loss of love for life. The newly evolved tension forces the individual to confront this inner conflict.

Two solutions exist: The individual is either ready to part with her strict principles to accept her needs and to face the challenges of daily life with all its necessary decision making or, in her efforts to avoid everything that does not fit her rigid principles, she enters the decompensation state, in which her principles degenerate into excess.

Crab Apple *(Malus pumila)*

Crab Apple types are conscientious and tidy. In their urge to be perfect they often fall into pedantry. The results are a fanatical tidiness and perfectionism. The Crab Apple type, however, lurks not only behind extremes like the compulsively clean housewife but also behind the harmless honor student who *must* complete his homework in an ideal manner. These people easily feel disgust not only for material objects such as dirt, bacteria, sweat, and excrement, which in their opinion are unclean, but also of "mental" dirt such as impure thoughts or bad moods. They are sensitive to any kind of disorder and find inner peace only when everything is in its proper place.

Crab Apple people say about themselves:

∾ I do everything very exactly, almost pedantically.

21

- I want to attract only positive attention.
- I am very painstaking in my job.
- I feel unclean if I cannot fulfill my own expectations.
- Everything has to be neat and perfect or else I create stress for myself. If I am not successful, I feel like a loser afterward.
- I often torture myself with little things and get stuck in details.
- I am very touchy about disorder. It really annoys me, in myself or in others.
- I am afraid of infections.
- I am disgusted by snakes and spiders.
- I take a shower at least once a day.
- Sometimes I even wash my hair twice a day.
- I am very fussy about cleanliness; it is almost a phobia.
- I can't use a toilet that is not mine; that is how disgusted I feel by it.
- I feel disgust for my own excrement and therefore do not like to eat because I don't want to digest.
- There are situations in which I feel I have to clean myself. Then I take shower or make myself vomit.
- When I eat too much or the wrong food, I put my finger down my throat to vomit. Otherwise I feel unclean.
- I feel that my body is unclean.
- I feel that sexuality is something dirty.
- I constantly try to defend myself against the negative and try not to get poisoned.
- I'm afraid of getting mentally infected by bad company.
- I don't want to have anything to do with drinkers or idlers.
- I feel internally unclean, especially after anger.

Crab Apple people have some points in common with Pines. Because the motivation in their states of mind is completely different, it is easy to differentiate between the two.

How does a person come to this extreme state of mind in which life becomes sterile because of fear of physical and mental infection?

We already saw how Rock Water people, afraid of betraying their own ideals, avoid everything that might lead them to immoral deeds. In extreme cases even contact with "unclean" people such as smokers, meat eaters, or "unbelievers" is avoided. Because they cannot simply shut off certain aspects of their personalities from life, they feel internally impure when they cannot adhere to their self-imposed prohibitions and when they go beyond their own narrow moral laws.

PINE TYPES	CRAB APPLE TYPES
Easily feel guilty	Feel internally unclean
Have a guilty conscience when they forget something; believe that they do not meet other people's expectations and are afraid of the consequences	Feel unworthy when they fail to live up to their own expectations
View sexuality as something that is forbidden	View sexuality as something morally bad and impure
	Have problems with everything concerning the body, such as kissing or nursing
Experience guilt and self-blame physically in the form of abdominal pain, lumbar pain, or headaches originating from the neck	Experience feelings of uncleanliness physically in the form of skin rashes, allergies, or bulimia

In time the feeling of being impure takes on a life of its own and is projected into all areas of life. The internal is transferred to the environment, where every form of impurity is fought against. Whatever we fight against in the external world, however, is really something that disturbs us about ourselves, as in the Hermetic law, "As above, so below."

If we reject the material, we also deny the spiritual principle behind it, whatever we choose to call it. Therefore, the dominant ideology in the Rock Water state questions itself in the Crab Apple state. The development from alienation from life in the Rock Water state to hostility against life in the Crab Apple State has led to a dead end. Those affected are continuously and simultaneously fighting on all levels against an environment they perceive as hostile. The physical embodiment of this defense is an allergy.

Crab Apple is used by many practitioners for eczema, allergies, and infected wounds, applying it topically in the form of compresses, ointments, or ointment dressings. For the prevention of infections or for already existing infections, it is also very useful.

Decompensation flower	Crab Apple
Compensation flower	Rock Water
Communication flower	Scleranthus

GENTIAN—WILLOW—WILD ROSE

Gentian *(Gentina amarella)*

Gentian people are eternal pessimists. They doubt everything and everyone and often even find a logical explanation for their negative attitude. Encountering external difficulties easily discourages them and makes them feel dejected. Because of their fear that something will go wrong anyway, they tend to give up easily, although it is just this negative expectation that thwarts success. When these people suffer setbacks in their family or career or in illnesses, their whole life falls apart. They cannot cope with even small difficulties and are often depressed about it.

Gentian people say about themselves:

- ∾ I question everything but rarely have a solution.
- ∾ It is difficult for me to see something in a positive light.
- ∾ I'm a pessimist.
- ∾ My common sense often tells me: "You must not believe everything."
- ∾ I can't trust and try to view everything realistically.
- ∾ I'm skeptical and say no first.
- ∾ I'm afraid that my trust will be abused and I'm therefore very careful.
- ∾ I worry constantly and brood: "What can you do better, how can you work better, what are you getting out of life?"
- ∾ I have often been disappointed by life. From these bad experiences I view everything in a negative way.
- ∾ It's hard for me to think positively about the future because I can't believe that my present situation will change.
- ∾ I get discouraged easily in difficult situations and doubt that they will turn out right.

Gentian people often give the impression that they are constantly looking for something negative, perhaps to justify their pessimistic attitude. One sometimes has the impression that these people actually do not like to feel good, because they hold on desperately to something negative and are always looking for the fly in the soup. On vacation it is often little things that spoil their fun. Sometimes they interpret something negative into it in retrospect to dampen their happiness and to justify their pessimistic attitude. Then, for example, they often say:

- ∾ It wasn't that great after all.
- ∾ It wasn't worth the money.
- ∾ The project wasn't worth the effort.
- ∾ We could have had that at home.
- ∾ Why did we drive all that way?

There are also Gentian types who can be recognized at a glance. They argue in the following way: "I see everything positively. Although there will be many difficulties and much annoyance, I am certain that I will succeed." The expectation of problems, however, is already a negative attitude, even if the person sets a positive goal and claims he is an optimist.

Another group of Gentians are people who point out over and over that they are critical and skeptical. There is often a hidden fear of appearing naive and gullible in our scientific society. Their supposed skeptisicm serves as self-protection and is meant to simulate strength. Their basic problem is a lack of self-esteem, which makes us think of the Larch flower. Nevertheless, those who constantly remind themselves to be skeptical will sooner or later turn into pessimists. Those who are skeptical from the very beginning make an objective examination difficult. It is better to be open to everything new and to form an opinion at the end, just as it is written in the Bible: "Examine everything, and keep the good."

The Gentian state can also appear as a result of a long-lasting illness, when the patient is frustrated and has doubts about the recovery. Where there are long-standing problems, marital conflicts, bad career situations in which there is no possibility for promotion or change, long-lasting unemployment, and other seemingly hopeless situations, one needs to consider Gentian. One has to differentiate, however, between doubt and frustration and resignation and inner capitulation.

Gentian is the remedy for exogenous reactive depression, that is, deep melancholy resulting from an event or an external situation. Gentian people should keep in mind that through their constantly negative thoughts they effectively create a cause that confirms their negative expectation—a self-fulfilling prophecy. Success is the result of positive thinking, failure the result of negative.

The perpetually gloomy outlook of these people wraps everything in dark clouds, and all the beauty of life stays hidden. All that is left is the void, which is the result of pessimistic thinking and not its cause. Gentian patients confuse cause and effect. Because everything in their lives seems to go wrong, it can easily happen that they feel like victims of their own fate. This leads to the decompensation state, in which they project the responsibility for their bad luck onto others.

Willow *(Salix vitellina)*

Willow people have already experienced a lot of bad luck in their lives. They see themselves as victims and always find a perpetrator for their bad luck, whether it be the neighbor, the vicious daughter-in-law, their own parents, the supervisor, or in extreme cases, the whole society or even destiny. They constantly believe that they are not treated fairly but instead of confronting their environment, they swallow their anger, fill up with bitterness, and withdraw more and more from life. Full of self-pity, they lament their alleged fate. The complaint, "What have I done to deserve this?" becomes their motto in life.

Willow people say about themselves:

- ∾ I feel unfairly treated.
- ∾ I often ask myself, "Why does it have to be me?" I am treated poorly by fate.
- ∾ I feel like a victim of destiny.
- ∾ I have never smoked, do not drink alcohol, and eat healthy. I often ask myself why it has to be me who is sick. How did I deserve this?
- ∾ Sometimes I envy other people's health.
- ∾ I turn my rage inward because it is not my style to argue with people.
- ∾ I often have to swallow my anger. That is why I am so bitter.
- ∾ I never forget how much pain somebody inflicted on me.
- ∾ I never have been able to forgive someone who hurt me.
- ∾ My rage is self-destructive. Once I even wanted to kill myself.
- ∾ I really wanted to learn a completely different job, but I didn't have the money for school. That is why my life is ruined.
- ∾ The doctors are to blame for my poor health. They recognized my disease too late.
- ∾ I can never be really happy.

In the Gentian state the affected persons constantly project the blame for their own bad luck onto other people. In this way they give up responsibility for their own fate. They do not want to see that they are the cause about which they now complain. Perhaps the reasons for their disappointment are too high expectations or the inability to accept the inevitable.

Those in the Willow state hold on to the negative. Sometimes one gets the feeling that they enjoy the role of the victim and the poorly treated. The expression of disapproval shows itself in frowns, which in time cause deep wrinkles in the corner of the mouth and the chin. Psychics report a dark aura with black spots in these bitter people. Their lives know only negativity. Even when these people appear nice on the outside under the surface lurk anger and bitterness. In contrast to the Holly types, however, this aggression does not reach the outside. Willow people do not explode or scold but rather seek their revenge by insulting the offender with taunting remarks. In the case of Holly the negative feelings are situation related and are ignited through an external event. For Willow, the negativism is a basic part of their personality.

Willow represents aggression, which goes inward and is focused on oneself—auto-aggression. The physical manifestation is rheumatism, in which antibodies that normally attack invading organisms destroy one's own body, especially the joints. The affected individuals painfully realize that they have to find the cause of their problems in themselves.

According to the law of cause and effect, the pessimistic attitude of the Gentian state, in which only negative things are expected, has brought bad luck upon itself. Instead of recognizing their mistakes, however, the individuals feel betrayed by their environment and their fate and retreat with bitter feelings. If it is not possible to stop this process of self-destruction, a state of decompensation will follow in which they will be crushed by their self-created suffering and give up inside.

Wild Rose *(Rosa canina)*

Wild Rose people have given up inside They are unhappy, unmotivated, and without any drive to change their situation. A Wild Rose state often appears in the following situations:

- An unsatisfying job
- A chronic illness
- An unhappy marriage
- An unwanted parenthood
- Imprisonment
- Poverty
- Wealth (bored with life)

Because these people can no longer imagine that their situation will ever change, they accept it without complaining and are indifferent and passive; they no longer show any interest in their surroundings. Nothing matters to them anymore, because they believe that everything is meaningless. They believe that their bad luck is predestined and illness hereditary or incurable, maybe even bad karma.

Wild Rose people say about themselves:

- ∾ Everything seems meaningless.
- ∾ I feel empty inside.
- ∾ Sometimes I'm completely apathetic, can't eat, can't work, can't be happy about anything.
- ∾ I have no desire for anything. There is nothing that makes me happy.
- ∾ I feel like I'm dead.
- ∾ I have no desire to live.
- ∾ I often think about suicide.
- ∾ I've given up on myself.
- ∾ I often feel emotionally drained and think, "I can't go on anymore. Everything is useless."

Wild Rose people have no drive or energy left, are constantly tired, and usually talk in a monotonous, expressionless voice. Their skin is pale and pasty; their blood pressure is very low and sometimes cannot be normalized even by blood pressure medication. In many cases they do not come to a practitioner of their own will but are brought by their relatives. Because they do not expect success in their therapy, they often ask, "What good will this do?"

There are, however, Wild Rose people who are not easily identified as such. Although they are active, they do not expect any more fulfillment from life. They work only out of a sense of duty and not with enjoyment (Oak component). Some can even move and inspire other people without being emotionally involved themselves (Vervain component). Others even appear happy on the outside and try to hide their inner emptiness from those around them (Agrimony component).

The Wild Rose state in some cases has already been overcome and yet is unconsciously present in everything they do. It is therefore important to ask in the intake interview if the patient has ever given up on life. This particular form of the Wild Rose state is not easily recognized. Extreme low blood pressure might be the key factor here. These people often feel more awake after the application of a few drops of the flower to the particular skin area. This is a good indicator of the Wild Rose state, even when the patients claim the state of resignation was many years ago. The skin zones provide a much more objective diagnosis than the interview. *New Bach Flower Body Maps* goes into more detail about this new form of Bach Flower Therapy.

Wild Rose is the result of the previous Willow state, even if this state lasted for only a short time. Prior to each resignation is the refusal to accept an external situation.

Whereas the embittered patient earlier withdrew himself, he now gives in

28

to his fate and fatalistically accepts it in the Wild Rose state because he has given up all hope. This makes <u>Wild Rose the strongest block in therapy.</u> It must not be overlooked, because otherwise every success in therapy—and not only in Bach Flower Therapy—will be questioned.

Decompensation flower	Wild Rose
Compensation flower	Willow
Communication flower	Gentian

WATER VIOLET—CHESTNUT BUD—BEECH

Water Violet *(Hottonia palustris)*

Water Violet types are independent and capable, well liked because of their superiority and tolerance. In problematic situations they stay cool, and their advice is in great demand because they stay objective and do not try to force their will on others. They do not interfere in other people's affairs, because they do not like it when other people try it on them.

The inner distance from their surroundings—which is highly regarded by others—can turn into a big problem in the long run however, because it is connected with a feeling of superiority. Confrontations are avoided not only because they are considered useless but also because they are beneath their dignity. In the long run these people discover that in many ways they really are superior to others. Because a tendency toward pride and arrogance already exists, they become more and more pretentious as a result. The feeling of being someone special develops, and consequently the inner distance from the surroundings becomes even greater.

Although Water Violet people are very much in demand and well liked in their career, they withdraw more and more into their private lives and even turn into loners and outsiders. They become even more unapproachable for others. This process creates loneliness and difficulties in making contact. As the ability to develop feelings of understanding, affection, or even love for their neighbors diminishes through an increase in arrogance, inner distance, and separation, it can lead to frigid feelings. This emotional state usually finds physical expression in spinal pain and a stiff neck, corresponding to a lack of humbleness and an inability to bend.

Water Violet people say about themselves:

- Sometimes I feel superior to others.
- Sometimes I'm arrogant toward other people.

∾ Other people think I am arrogant.

∾ I always have been the best, in school, in college, in my job. My motto is: "I never fail."

∾ I often feel isolated, and I seek distance.

∾ I have more experience than others.

∾ I have the feeling that there are more dormant ideas and abilities in me than in other people.

∾ I would rather do things myself because others can't do it as well as I can.

∾ I don't like to be helped, but I like to help other people.

∾ I don't let other people do my work, because then I would have to thank them.

∾ I don't like it when other people interfere in my affairs.

∾ I often feel superior inside. Sometimes that feels embarrassing, sometimes it feels nice.

∾ I always try to act very distinguished.

∾ I don't want to have anything to do with certain people.

∾ It's hard to be subordinate to other people, even to my supervisor.

∾ I'm afraid to live an average life and to float along.

∾ I have problems with humbleness.

A Water Violet state often is present in aristocrats as a result of their elitist upbringing. People with exceptional abilities (gifted children, geniuses, successful people) are also predisposed to this particular state of mind, as are people with special qualities (for example, extraordinarily beautiful people, models, or body builders). Those in certain professions, such as artists, actors, and politicians, who are popular and carry an image of celebrity, are easily enticed to really feel superior. These people often try to do everything perfectly, to distinguish themselves even more from the rest. Götz Blome writes: "Pride needs admirers and destroys the innocent nature of every quality. . . . It creates hierarchies and separates us from other people. . . . pride is an inhumane quality. It shows that we have forgotten how to be human and how to rise above this. . . . It prevents us from thinking, talking, or acting in a friendly way and creates a barrier between us and others."[2]

If this feeling of superiority is not stopped Water Violet people are in danger of feeling superior to things that in their eyes are completely unimportant and banal. In this way they walk right by the most important tasks and lessons of life and avoid everything unpleasant in the state of compensation because it is in their opinion beneath their dignity.

Chestnut Bud *(Aesculus hippocastanum)*

People who need Chestnud Bud do not learn easily from their mistakes. Through their ignorant and superficial manner they miss out on many things in life and compulsively make the same mistakes over and over again. These can be little things like:

- ∾ Forgetting their keys
- ∾ Not turning off the stove
- ∾ Always taking the right of way from someone at an intersection
- ∾ Not being able to turn off the TV at night and then going to work the next morning completely tired
- ∾ Eating sweets immediately after a diet and then being upset about the newly regained weight
- ∾ Having a drag of a cigarette after quitting smoking and then starting all over again
- ∾ Always getting fooled by the same type of salesperson
- ∾ Always buying the same type of used car despite expensive repairs in the past

These people constantly repeat their mistakes in more important areas of their lives as well. For example, again and again they have affairs with someone who is married, although they have suffered many times before in these relationships. Or they start a new area of study without ever completing one.

Chestnut Bud people say about themselves:

- ∾ I sometimes make it very easy on myself.
- ∾ I avoid problems as a matter of principle.
- ∾ I put off work until the very last minute.
- ∾ I start to dawdle if a job is boring to me.
- ∾ I like to postpone unpleasant tasks and am happy when something else comes up.
- ∾ I often fiddle around and finish up thousands of unimportant tasks just to avoid the main task.
- ∾ I often make the same mistake.
- ∾ I sometimes lose my train of thought and don't remember what I wanted to do or say.
- ∾ On vacation I always order the same soup in the same restaurant from the same waiter, although I was very angry the last time to have been served diluted ketchup as tomato soup.

- ∾ I am always late for my appointments. If I set the alarm half an hour earlier, I somehow fiddle around so much that I end up being in a hurry.
- ∾ I constantly buy books, but only flip the pages without reading them.
- ∾ I tape all the interesting movies from TV, but I've rarely watched any of them.
- ∾ I become enthusiastic very fast, but the initial euphoria fades away quickly like a castle in the air.
- ∾ I read many books simultaneously because I lose the initial fascination with a book after a short time and then become interested in another book.
- ∾ I often start many things at the same time but do not complete them.
- ∾ In my thoughts I am always two steps ahead and think about what I will do next. Therefore, I'm often distracted from my current task.
- ∾ I make many plans for the future.
- ∾ I often act against my own inner voice, even when I know from the start that it will go wrong.

This state of mind often expresses itself in chronic physical complaints, as if the affected person needs to repeat the same mistake inside the body. Some Chestnut Bud patients show symptoms of illness that correspond to their emotional conflicts. Their problems in walking show symbolically that they constantly want to run away from something.

Typically, these people can become euphoric about some things, but are not very interested in the affairs of daily life. They carve out highly ambitious plans and are already deliberating over their next project, although they have not even started with their current work. For this reason they are unfocused, forgetful, and do not conduct their work accurately. They often start many things at the same time and do not finish them.

They put unpleasant and momentarily uninteresting things aside to finish them up later, when they feel like doing them. For example, one can always find their stack of magazines and books that they started to read and want to finish later. They often occupy their time with unimportant little things to justify the neglect of their real work. If they are confronted with this, they always find a convincing and logical explanation for it. They often argue that it is the workload that keeps them from doing their job.

The behavior of Chestnut Bud people is influenced by their evasion of everything unpleasant and uninteresting. Driven internally like a rocket, they constantly plunge into new experiences, have thousands of ideas in their heads, and create new plans for the future, but live in an inner haste. Their self-inflicted sensory overload leads to a lack of concentration, memory problems, and the inability to keep up with the tasks of daily life, all of which make them feel indifferent and lose interest in the present situation. In comparison to Clematis people, who live in a dream world full of fantasies and castles in the air, their attention is captured by concrete things and realistic ideas. Honeysuckle people also live in a world full of thoughts, but they dwell in the past, which they long to go back to because it awakens pleasant memories inside them.

Chestnut Bud is the sequel to Water Violet. Whereas the Water Violet person withdraws from everything *internally* because she thinks it is below her dignity, the Chestnut Bud person distances herself *externally* from it as well, by repressing everything unpleasant and ugly and postponing least favorite work until the very last.

The fact that she makes the same mistakes again and again, however, shows that the lessons of life cannot be completely put aside. It will therefore come to a state of decompensation, if the individual is not willing to confront her own mistakes. Again, she will confront her environment, but by seeking the mistakes in others.

Beech *(Fragus sylvatica)*

Beech people are notorious grumblers. Because they look everywhere for the negative, they almost always find a fly in the soup. Empathy, tolerance, and understanding for the little mistakes of other people are unknown to them. On the contrary, they are strict and often complain about little things. Especially typical for them is the angry complaint: "How could you?" Frowning to express their displeasure, they are viewed as arrogant. Because of their barbed wit and cynical criticism, their popularity decreases more and more. Other people often withdraw from them, because they feel insulted by the constant condescension.

Beech people say about themselves:

- I like to criticize.
- I'm not able to keep my mouth shut when there are obvious wrongs, even if this makes me unpopular.
- I often find fault.
- Other people call me a nag.
- I criticize other people only for their own good and because I want to help them by pointing out their mistakes to them.
- I'm often bothered by other people's superficiality.
- I tend to put down the thoughts of others.
- I tend to make ironic comments and tease.

- ∾ I sometimes am very proud of myself when I'm able to characterize a miserable situation with the right words.
- ∾ I would have been a good satirist.
- ∾ The laugh is always on the losers.
- ∾ My sarcastic kind of humor is often insulting to others.
- ∾ Friends tell me my biting humor is disgusting.
- ∾ I think that those who cannot laugh about other people's mistakes are losers.
- ∾ It is the person's own fault if he can't take criticism and feels insulted by my friendly teasing.
- ∾ I don't understand why some people are so sensitive and react so allergically to a little criticism.
- ∾ I don't like it if someone is nagging me for no reason. I criticize only when it is absolutely necessary and serves a good purpose.

The Beech state indicates that the individual is already in a phase of decompensation. This problem must be treated immediately, even if the patient thinks that this flower is not important and they would rather exchange it for another one.

A Beech state is a deeply rooted flaw in the personality. By vehemently fighting the little mistakes of others in a self-satisfied way, those afflicted divert themselves from their own problems because they refuse to face their own imperfection. Whereas during the Water Violet state these people thought that they performed perfectly the tasks they considered important, in the Chestnut Bud state they are forced to realize that they often made the same mistakes over and over again, esspecially in the simple tasks of life.

In the Beech state they now look for the mistakes in other people, to distract themselves from their own imperfections, which insult their arrogance and pride and disturb their inner feeling of superiority. The realization that they have not learned enough from their own mistakes is easier to handle if these mistakes can also be found in other people. The tendency toward insolence and pride, coupled with the compulsive search for mistakes in other people, ultimately leads to arrogance and intolerance. The individuals might not be troubled by this attitude and therefore not aware of the problem, because they always excuse the complaints with the "oversensitiveness" of others. This makes itself more painfully present in the physical domain, however, because in time the intolerant state of mind extends itself to the body, which defends itself vehemently against small things and toxins such as pollen, house dust, and feathers. The "allergy" against the shortcomings of other people has thereby manifested itself.

It has now become necessary to admit to oneself and to others the mistake one has made and to come down off one's high horse. Otherwise, this wrong behavior will not only get unpleasant but also dangerous in time. Just as nagging and criticizing is viewed as an assault and therefore threatening to the personality, the allergy can become life threatening in its extreme form as anaphylactic shock.

Decompensation flower	Beech
Compensation flower	Chestnut Bud
Communication flower	Water Violet

VERVAIN—HORNBEAM—CHESTNUT
∾

Vervain *(Verbena officinalis)*

Vervain types are enthusiastic and idealistic. They want to share their ideas and experiences with others and try to move others with passionate speeches. They feel disappointed and dejected if they are unsuccessful and set their minds to coming up with new words that may yet convince others.

The constant effort to convert other people does not let them rest internally and causes them to overwork themselves to the point of exhaustion. For this reason they are always tense and have problems falling asleep. In their desire to convince the world of something they often overdo it and appear to be fanatic, inflexible, and dogmatic. They are often engaged in never-ending discussions and easily end up in conflict because they are unyielding in their point of view and even try to force their convictions on their opponent. They sometimes even believe they are chosen by fate to enlighten others. To other people their missionary passion appears tiring and exhausting, which means they are avoided.

Vervain people say about themselves:

- ∾ When I feel enthusiastic about something, I immediately have to tell someone about it.
- ∾ When someone does not listen to me it drives me crazy.
- ∾ When I have a good idea I want to pass it on immediately.
- ∾ I constantly try to convince people of my ideas, even when they don't show interest in them. I often feel completely exhausted afterward but can't go to sleep because I feel so tense.
- ∾ I can stand up for something with all my energy and conviction.

- I have strong ideals. If I am convinced about something, I can fight for it to the bitter end.
- The worst thing for me is wanting to say something and not being allowed to do so.
- I can't bear injustice.
- I have high expectations of myself.
- I want to do everything perfectly.
- I want to be faultless.
- I try to electrify other people.
- I want to influence people in a positive way, and if necessary I use force.
- It is easy for me to convince other people.
- I set goals in my life and don't rest until I have achieved them.
- I do everything absolutely accurately. Although I expect myself to be this way, I don't care about it in other people.
- I suffer from stress and can't relax.
- My biggest problem is my inner tension. I always feel tense somewhere.

The quest for perfection in Vervain has an entirely different character from the one in Crab Apple. Crab Apple personalities perform all of the tasks they are given accurately and conscientiously. They act out of an inner obsession in a pedantic manner, because otherwise they would feel impure. Vervain types, on the other hand, are inspired by an idea in which they engage themselves completely. Other things are trivialities to which they do not pay much attention.

Whereas Crab Apple students get good grades in all their classes, Vervain students try to obtain high grades in only one or two classes and to break all the records in them. In other classes they are average because they are not interested in the topics. It is also possible for a Vervain student to fail all his classes because he has a hobby that absorbs all his attention. Vervain students attract attention in the classroom because they do not usually raise their hands when they have something to say but instead snap their fingers, interrupt, and do not rest until their message gets across. Vervain adults can be a real nuisance for public speakers with their statements and strong opinions. Afterward, they apologize with the statement, "I just had to get it off my chest."

The difference between Vervain and Rock Water people is that the latter try to embody a certain ideal or ideology to prove its practical application, whereas Vervain people only try to prove themselves. Mediocrity is unbearable to them. The physical consequences of this constant mental strain show themselves in states of internal and external tension, for example:

- Muscle tension
- High blood pressure
- Spasms and colics
- Headaches
- Hyperactivity and the inability to relax
- The constant feeling of being stressed
- Nervousness and nervous ticks
- Inner restlessness

These people often have an overactive thyroid gland. The Vervain state can lead—as a result of constant mental depletion—to a compensatory Hornbeam state.

Hornbeam *(Carpininus betulus)*

People who need Hornbeam feel overwhelmed by life. They believe that they are unable to withstand the challenges of daily life, feel weak, are without energy, and suffer under a great deal of mental fatigue. Every day feels like a Monday morning, and they like to stay in bed as long as possible. The longer they stay in bed, the more exhausted they feel. The thought of work makes them even weaker. Oddly enough, their work proceeds very well once they have started it.

Hornbeam people say about themselves:

- Lately I've been competely exhausted.
- I'm tired and would prefer to lie in bed all day.
- I've been overworking myself lately.
- I wake up in the morning more tired than when I went to bed the night before.
- I only have to think about my work and I become more and more tired. It takes a great deal of convincing to get started. But the more I work the easier it gets.
- My work doesn't come easy these days. Just the thought of how much I have to do on a particular day makes me feel dreadful.
- I don't feel strong enough for my work.
- I often feel drained inside.
- I often lose my concentration.

∾ I have a difficult time thinking.

∾ I hang around for hours sometimes before I can get myself to do something.

∾ When I work or watch TV until late at night, my eyes start burning and watering because they feel weak.

The Hornbeam state is the result of a singular mental strain that is constantly practiced by people of the Vervain type. An excess of mental work without physical compensation, for example by students, secretaries, and managers, creates an imbalance between the mental and the physical realm. As a consequence the brain virtually shuts down to force the individual to reestablish a harmony between the two levels. A Hornbean state should therefore be an alarm signal for the person concerned.

Hornbeam shows certain similarities to Elm, Olive, and Larch and therefore has to be carefully distinguished from those states. Larch people also feel overwhelmed; however, it is not weakness or overexertion but lack of self-esteem that makes these individuals doubt their own abilities. Olive people are in a state of total physical and emotional exhaustion, in which they have become incapable of performing any task. Hornbeam patients, in contrast, feel temporarily strained and state that they cannot cope at this particular moment but would be able to with more strength or after a good night's sleep.

An Elm state occurs in rather acute situations in which the individuals are burdened with too many demands and expectations, such as examinations. Those tasks stand before them like an insurmountable wall. They do not lack strength, as with Hornbeam or Olive, but only stamina.

An unrecognized Hornbeam state can extend into a White Chestnut state, the state of decompensation.

White Chestnut *(Aesculus hippocastanum)*

It is difficult for White Chestnut people to unwind. Their thoughts are constantly spinning around in their heads, and they are unable to fight it. Because the thoughts repeat themselves over and over again, they cannot find rest and go over their problems without finding a solution. This produces headaches, lack of concentration, tightness in the forehead, eye pain, and inner agitation and nervousness.

White Chestnut people say about themselves:

∾ It's hard for me to wind down.

∾ I often talk to myself.

∾ I can't concentrate because there are thousands of thoughts going through my head.

- ∞ I often remember unpleasant situations, which come back to bother me again.
- ∞ I often try to push my thoughts aside, but I am not able to. It seems that they follow me everywhere.
- ∞ I frequently remember embarrassing situations and I would like to run away from myself. Even when I convince myself that the situation is long past, I still can't get it out of my mind.
- ∞ I still think about conversations that I had a long time ago. It always makes me angry when I think about what I forgot to say.
- ∞ Often I continue with discussions in my mind and think about what I should have said.
- ∞ For hours I can't get it out of my mind when someone has made me angry. Sometimes this goes on in my head for days, and I think about how I could have defended myself better.
- ∞ I'm always noticing another thing in our house that we could have done differently when we built it. Because of that, I can't enjoy the house the way it is now. In my head I constantly plan how it could be better, although the house was finished a long time ago.
- ∞ I wish I could just switch off these constant thoughts and find peace inside myself.
- ∞ I don't sleep well because I can't turn off my thoughts.
- ∞ I'm constantly tired.

White Chestnut has a certain similarity to Clematis and Honeysuckle. Based on different objectives, however, it is easy to distinguish the flowers from each other. Clematis people are always thinking, yet theirs are pleasant thoughts and daydreams, in which the individual dwells voluntarily, whereas thoughts in the White Chestnut case are useless and even annoying. White Chestnut individuals would be happy if they could rid themselves of these compulsive thoughts. Honeysuckle people also live in a world of thought, but it is the past into which they escape. They dwell in pleasant memories of the good old times.

White Chestnut is often used in combination with Pine, Gentian, or Star of Bethlehem. In coexisting Pine states, thoughts are colored with guilty feelings and self-accusation. The affected person often thinks: "I should have . . . !" When White Chestnut is used in combination with Gentian, thoughts are of a brooding nature, accompanied by worries and pessimistic impulses. If the White Chestnut state appears in combination with the Star of Bethlehem state, an earlier emotional trauma is forcing itself back into consciousness. Old unpleasant events surface again, constantly burdening the individual.

White Chestnut emerges as the result of preceding Vervain and Hornbeam states. While people in the Vervain state exhaust themselves with their colossal enthusiasm, as a result they suffer under mental fatigue and weakness. Consequently, a yin state compensates for a highly strung yang state. The affected person acts passively and in extreme cases spends the entire day in bed.

Whereas the body has already been neglected in the Vervain state as a result of an overemphasis on the intellectual, both physical and mental activity is now reduced in the Hornbeam state because of mental weakness. But the body is unable to be inactive for even one second of its life—the heart is beating around the clock. Therefore, activity has to happen, in this case the intellectual kind. According to the same mechanism, people who sleep long have difficulty going to sleep at night.

The Hornbeam phase can sometimes be of short duration. It is often even bypassed through stimulating substances like coffee, black tea, cola, and nicotine. These substances take the White Chestnut state into the phase of decompensation. Coffee is known to cause sleeplessness through chasing one's own thoughts.

To get out of the decompensation phase it is necessary to stop neglecting the body. Not only physical activities such as jogging and bicycling but also saunas, dry brushing, and cold rubdowns can be very beneficial. Especially the latter can eliminate tormenting thoughts if done just before bedtime and facilitate a deep and refreshing sleep.

Decompensation flower	White Chestnut
Compensation flower	Hornbeam
Communication flower	Vervain

AGRIMONY—VERVAIN—SWEET CHESTNUT

ॐ

Agrimony *(Agrimonia eupatoria)*

Agrimony people always seem cheerful and lighthearted. They are always in a good mood and up for a good joke, are pleasant companions, and are liked everywhere because they create a pleasant atmosphere. Their cheerfulness is so contagious that others are hardly ever bored in their presence.

This easiness however is a facade behind which deep agony is hidden. Tortured by worries, cares, and fears, they seek the company of others to forget their problems. Because they do not want to burden others with their problems, however, they try to downplay them or hide them. In this way they continuously run away from themselves and need excitement and activity to deal with their fears.

On principle they avoid conflicts and arguments, because they are extremely sensitive and peace loving. Most of all they suffer a great deal under disharmony and discord.

Agrimony people say about themselves:

- I don't want to burden other people with my problems and therefore keep them to myself.
- I solve my problems on my own and don't show them to the outside. Instead I listen to music or read a book and try to distract myself.
- I'm afraid to open myself up to others.
- I hide a lot. I didn't tell anyone about my illness.
- I'm afraid to reveal myself to others.
- I share very little about my problems. I keep the main things to myself.
- I have to feel extremely bad before I'll admit it.
- At work I put on a mask, which sometimes feels like a wall.
- I live according to the principle "Keep smiling" because I was raised that way.
- I can fool people by hiding my fears.
- Even in my psychotherapy I covered up a lot at first.
- In the past I always pretended to be a happy person and went to many parties; internally, however, I had given up. At night in my sleep I was grinding my teeth.
- I don't let anyone get close to me.
- I'm afraid to have closer contact and therefore keep things rather superficial.
- I don't like to admit my feelings to other people.
- I conceal a lot, because I had to hide a lot in the past.
- I can't show happiness in the right way.
- I've tried to help other people so I could run away from my own feelings and needs.
- When I hold back my feelings, I stop breathing and I can't take a deep breath.

The Agrimony state is easily overlooked because those affected are not truthful even to the people to whom they turn for help. In the interview they evade questions or trivialize their problems. Statements that point toward problems are contradicted in the following sentence or are described with expressions like "maybe," "perhaps," or "I'm inclined to think . . ." When they talk about their problems at all, it is only superficially. They try to downplay their illness and poke fun at serious findings.

In a physical exam one notices that acupuncture points that should be pressure sensitive according to the complaints and laboratory findings do not respond at all. The principle of repression has already moved from the emotional realm to the body, so that it is impossible to recognize disturbances through its alarm points.

The emotional pressure on these people and the inner restlessness express themselves often through nervous finger drumming, trembling of the hands, nervous tics, or nighttime teeth grinding. They have problems falling asleep at night because everything they have repressed during the day comes to the surface. The longer they lie in bed, the more restless they become. To escape their tormenting thoughts, they stay up late at night watching TV, reading, or trying other activities to distract themselves. They are very susceptible to alcohol and pharmaceutical and other drugs, because these things help them forget their fears.

Gentian people are tormented by worries as well, but they create these worries themselves by holding on to negativism. They constantly complain about their problems, whereas Agrimony people repress everything negative and try to ignore their problems. Yet the problems cannot be completely driven out of the consciousness and reappear like a boomerang again and again. The more they try to push away their sorrows, the bigger the inner counterpressure will be. The affected individuals thereupon escape even more into the external world and need more and more action to avoid their thoughts.

Because the outer image has to withstand this inner pressure, these individuals will tense up more and more. As a consequence physical symptoms start to develop that symbolize a holding on, for example, constipation or a nervous bladder. In this latter case only a certain portion will be released with urination, while the rest will be retained in the bladder. Painful urination also indicates that the process of letting go is experienced as something painful.

Without knowing it, Agrimony people often have problems making contact. Their relationships are superficial because they keep other people at a distance from themselves. They are unable to have deeper emotional contact because they are afraid to reveal too much about themselves.

On the other hand, because they need acquaintanceships to distract themselves from their fears and sorrows and are actually dependent on them, they look for contacts but simultaneously keep a fearful inner distance. They are afraid of real emotions, because these emotions could threaten their superficial relationship with their "friends." Anyone who always hides his feelings from the outside world runs the risk of not knowing himself anymore.

The outer facade becomes the alter ego, with whom over time one will identify to such a degree that the awareness about oneself—about one's real feelings and needs—will eventually be lost.

Because of this build-up of painful pressure, the personality must find a way to release this inner tension. The simplest solution is to let go; that, however, is the most difficult task these individuals can imagine. This possibility cannot be achieved without help; therefore, the stage of compensation follows, in which the escape to the outside world is pursued by even more extreme means: By attempting to interest others in ideas or ideals, these individuals think they can distract themselves and others from themselves.

Agrimony is the most difficult flower to diagnose. It is often impossible to draw conclusions from the statements of the patients; one must rely on one's own ability to observe. People who complain about inner restlessness but appear to be calm on the outside, as well as children whose tears dry up quickly and who soon become cheerful again and cope with unpleasant situations surprisingly well, should be considered for Agrimony. Chronic obesity or yo-yo dieting also indicates that an emotional conflict is compensated for by eating. Agrimony people generally have some kind of hidden vice.

A state of Agrimony is often the result of an acute crisis, for example, the death of a relative or the separation from a partner who has found a new lover, and it represents the individual's processing of the conflict. The crisis may be found in childhood, for example, when parents did not spent enough time with the affected individual, therefore he had to learn to work things out for himself. Children sometimes adopt the behavior pattern of the parents. The phrase "Big boys don't cry" indicates a repression of feelings.

In principle, however, one can assume that a certain predisposition for this kind of attitude existed previously and the corresponding situation functioned only as a trigger. The horoscope can be of real help in recognizing this state more clearly. In such a case one should pay especially close attention to the ascendant and the position of the moon. In therapy-resistant cases Agrimony is also worth a try, because it brings repressed feelings to the surface.

Vervain *(Verbena officinalis)*

The Vervain state reappears here as the compensation for the Agrimony state. The symptoms are the same as described above for the track of Vervain—Hornbeam—White Chestnut. The difference, though, is the motivation that has led to this state and, accordingly, the way in which it is compensated or decompensated.

Vervain is used as a communication flower when those afflicted exaggerate in their excitement and try to influence others with their ideas. In their zeal they exploit their own energies. This leads to a state of exhaustion, which forces the individuals to take it easier in the compensation state. But when the Vervain state occurs as compensation for the Agrimony state, those afflicted become overactive to hide their innermost selves. Through an excessively extroverted lifestyle it is possible for them to distract themselves from their emotional pain, sorrows, and fears. If an external calamity is added to the internal misery, then—literally—enough is enough, and they are no longer able to hide their problems; on the contrary, blocked emotions accumulated over the years increase the emotional pain. They react with a state of deep despair, in which they think they will be broken by their fate.

Sweet Chestnut *(Castanea sativa)*

People who need Sweet Chestnut are absolutely despondent. An unexpected blow or a seemingly hopeless situation has brought them to the limit of their emotional endurance. They do not know what to do anymore because they have already tried everything. In this way they experience the sudden pointlessness of their former actions. This total hopelessness leads to a state of deepest despair and inner void, in which they even feel deserted by God and no longer know hope. They can neither pray nor cry, and they fear that their fate is breaking down.

Sweet Chestnut people say about themselves:

- ∾ I feel absolute despair.
- ∾ I don't see any way out of this situation.
- ∾ I can't bear this situation any longer.
- ∾ I can neither laugh nor cry anymore; I feel a complete void inside of me, and I don't know what more I can do.
- ∾ I've tried everything, and now I feel completely hopeless.
- ∾ I can't stand it any longer, otherwise I will breakdown.
- ∾ God has abandoned me.

People in a Sweet Chestnut state keep their pain to themselves, similar to those in the Agrimony state, whereas Gorse people wail about their suffering to everyone. They keep their emotions under control in even the most extreme cases of emotional suffering in contrast to Cherry Plum people, who are capable of committing suicide when they snap. A debate with and a desperate fight against irrevocable fate still takes place in Sweet Chestnut people. In the Wild Rose state, on the other hand, the individuals have given up and even consider suicide as an alternative to the hopelessness of their situation. This would be planned very carefully, whereas in the Cherry Plum State it would occur completely unsuspected by others.

In sudden strokes of fate, such as the death of a close relative, the Sweet Chesnut state appears rather suddenly, seemingly without preexisting problems of any kind. This is actually not the case, however. The nature of people determines how they will react in extreme emotional situations. If they repress negativity (Agrimony) they will despair (Sweet Chestnut). If they hold on to negativity (Gentian), they will resist against their fate (Willow), but give up with increasing emotional pressure (Wild Rose).

Extreme emotional situations bring hidden and latent emotional conflicts to the surface of the consciousness by catapulting the individual without prior warning into the phase of decompensation. Therefore, it is important to activate the hidden flower concepts behind the problems as soon as the patient gets over the initial crisis, because the real problem cannot be solved with situation-related flower remedies.

Decompensation flower	Sweet Chestnut
Compensation flower	Vervain
Communication flower	Agrimony

ROCK ROSE—AGRIMONY—CHERRY PLUM

Rock Rose (Helianthemum nummularium)

The Rock Rose flower is used in extreme emotional situations, in crises, and in external circumstances that produce fear and horror for the individual. The following situations often lead to acute Rock Rose states.

- Accidents
- A devastating blow, such as the death of a family member
- Severe terminal illness, such as heart attacks or strokes
- Traumatic experiences, for example, when a mouse jumps into one's face in a pitch black basement
- Life-threatening situations, such as near drowning, car accidents, or suffocation attacks

In those situations the affected individuals experience feelings of:

- Panic
- Terror
- Sheer horror
- Being scared to death

~ Being paralyzed from fear
~ Being unable to think straight
~ Being totally powerless
~ Sensing one's heart has stopped beating

They often describe these situations with the words, "It hit me like lightning."

The following physical symptoms can appear: paralysis, sudden loss of hearing or speech, feelings of being ice cold, shaking, loss of control.

The Rock Rose state occurs only in acute situations. There are Rock Rose types who are inclined to deal with unpleasant situations by going into shock. They are very sensitive, panic easily, and are susceptible to neuroses and disturbances of the nervous system. Some authors connect this with a hormonal disorder of the suprarenal gland. The fear in these people is not a chronic state as it is, for example, in Mimulus and Aspen types. Most of the time they do not appear to be frightened. One has the impression that a hidden fear that is deeply rooted in the subconscious becomes frequently reactivated by external events.

Where does this fear come from? One interpretation is offered by therapies in which it is possible to relive one's own birth. It is often observed that feelings of panic and fear caused by complications during delivery are still stored in the subconscious and are relived again with the same intensity during therapy. Even after so many years they seem not to have lost any of their original dramatic quality. The disorders that are apparently connected to the birth experience often disappear completely after these feelings are experienced once more and integrated into the conscious mind.

One female patient experienced her panic again with rebirthing (a therapy in which the breathing rhythm of a newborn baby is imitated to trigger memories of birth); during her birth the umbilical cord had been wrapped around her neck. After several rebirthing sessions her chronic headaches disappeared. Interestingly enough, she also suffered from occasional nightmares and nocturnal states of mind that are reminiscent of the birth experience. She reported, "I suffer sometimes from nocturnal attacks of suffocation. Something is compressing my throat. Then I always panic and become so confused that I can't find the light switch and desperately try to find my way in the dark. I often have no idea where I am."

Perhaps the nightmares from which Rock Rose people often awake screaming are memories of repressed experiences that thrust themselves back into the consciousness in a dream. These traumatic experiences must go back very far, because the patients are not aware of them anymore. The cause is often the birth experience, as the above therapies show. Because every birth is traumatic in some way—we will refer to this later in conjunction with the

Star of Bethlehem—many therapists give the Star of Bethlehem as the first Bach Flower Remedy. If there was a fear of death at birth, Rock Rose should be given instead.

We should keep in mind that the umbilical cord is cut soon after delivery in almost every birth clinic, an unhealthy custom that except in "easy delivery" is still widely practiced today. The newborn baby is scared to death when the umbilical cord is cut before it starts to breath on its own. It has to breathe immediately or else it will die. One can see this fear of dying on many babies' faces. The first breath of life is accompanied by a fearful cry that is interpreted as a sign that the baby is well. If it does not breathe immediately, it receives the famous "slap on the butt."

So formed, this Rock Rose state will remain largely undetected. Nightmares might be understood as a vague hint, but the precise symptoms for diagnosing this flower remedy are often missing.

Agrimony *(Agrimony eupatoria)*

The Agrimony state occurs here as the compensation for a previously occurring Rock Rose state. The fear and the memories of a possibly preexisting trauma are repressed. In the Agrimony state as described in the track of Agrimony-Vervain-Sweet Chestnut, individuals try to hide their emotional problems from the outside and feign cheerfulness and lightheartedness. The flower picture in both cases is the same. The repression of unpleasant things is acted out on different levels, however: in the case of compensation, primarily in the confrontation with one's own psyche; in the other case, through interaction with one's surroundings. For this reason the individuals are even less aware of their compensation state and therefore even harder for the therapist to recognize.

Many times this inner conflict—triggered by an experience of extreme panic or deadly fear—will be visible in the phase of decompensation. Here the repressed contents of the conscious mind push themselves with force back to the surface and create a panicky fear in the individuals that the tools of repression will fail and they will lose control.

Because the Agrimony state functions as a protection against one's subconscious conflicts that are viewed as threatening, one should prescribe Agrimony very carefully and closely watch the reaction of the patient after application. It is possible that the repressed unconscious material will return to the individual's consciousness in the form of dreams, relived fears, or even clear memories. If after the application of Agrimony an inner agitation appears that could eventually increase in force, the application of the flower should be stopped for a while and the decompensation flower given, even when it does not seem to fit the symptoms.

Cherry Plum *(Prunnus cerasifera)*

People who need Cherry Plum have the feeling that they have a time bomb inside that could explode at any moment. They are afraid of their own feelings and fear that if they let them go a terrible disaster will happen.

Their fear of going crazy or wild drives them to the brink of desperation. In this extreme emotional state they are afraid of losing control of themselves and committing terrible atrocities against their will. In their obsessions they imagine how they would kill other people in a brutal way or how they would do themselves harm. The fear of turning these crazy notions into action makes them almost lose their minds. They believe that they will go crazy and fear a nervous breakdown or being committed to a psychiatric clinic.

People who need Cherry Plum say about themselves:

- ∾ I'm afraid of losing my self-control, afraid that I will freak out.
- ∾ I'm afraid of losing my mind.
- ∾ I can't let go internally.
- ∾ When stress gets to be too much, I'm afraid of losing control of myself.
- ∾ I often think, "What are you doing now? What will happen if you go crazy now?"
- ∾ I'm afraid that the violence in myself will break out.
- ∾ I'm afraid that someday I would be able to kill my grandmother.
- ∾ I'm tormented by the delusion of throwing my child out the window. I know I would normally never do this, but I'm terribly afraid that someday I won't be able to resist this inner force and will act out this horrible delusion.
- ∾ I've never been able to let go completely, have never lost my temper, but when I keep myself under control I get migraines. When I was a child my mother had serious heart disease. My father always told me, "Be quiet, otherwise mother will get very sick."
- ∾ I often have the feeling that I would lose my mind if something happened to the children.
- ∾ I'm afraid of myself, of my own feelings, of the dark feelings deep inside of me.
- ∾ During meditation everything suddenly turns pitch black and I can see grimaces; then I have to stop.
- ∾ I often suffer from emotional agony. Inside of me is a wrenching desire for the redemption of my soul.

During a simple relaxation exercise a patient once told me, "I can't close my eyes for fear that I'll lose control. I'm afraid that something psychic will happen that I won't be able to undo later."

A Cherry Plum state is the result of a prior Agrimony state. In the Agrimony state unpleasant things are repressed; in the Cherry Plum state this repressed matter causes fear. In its acute form it occurs mainly as a result of drug consumption. This state can sometimes exist for years after the last dose of drugs. Such persons are often noticable because they cannot even wait for five minutes for fear they will go crazy. They would rather take a short walk.

An acquaintance of mine fell into such a state as a result of taking LSD and could no longer stand any kind of monotonous noise. Especially while riding the bus it became a problem. The bus had to stop sometimes in the middle of the road for him, and he had to walk for miles, because he was convinced that the engine noise would make him lose his mind. At the time, I did not use Bach Flowers but I was able to help him let go with the help of a simple meditative exercise. He immediately lost his fear and told me later that shortly after the exercise he took the bus home and even enjoyed the ride.

Cherry Plum people have to learn to let go from within. Because they fearfully repress all the impulses originating in their subconsciousness, counterpressure builds up from within, violently pushing the repressed experiences and dark sides of the personality back to the surface of consciousness. Unwanted confrontation with one's own shadow creates intense fear. If Cherry Plum individuals learn to endure these surfacing images and impressions and do not offer any resistance, the scare fades away quickly. By fighting against it they maintain the situation. Everything we fight returns to haunt us.

A Cherry Plum state is not always as acute as described above. Under certain circumstances it feeds on itself for years. In these cases there is typically an inner force that the individual cannot pull away from. Cherry Plum is used in such cases in combination with other flowers. The following are suitable for:

Compulsive cleaning	Crab Apple
The urge to smile all the time	Agrimony
Compulsive criticizing and lecturing	Beech
Inability to wind down; constant thinking	White Chestnut
Paranoia with compulsive behavior	Aspen
Compulsive questioning	Cerato

ॐ

Decompensation flower	Cherry Plum
Compensation flower	Agrimony
Communication flower	Rock Rose

IMPATIENS—OLIVE—OAK

∾

Impatiens *(Impatiens glandulifera)*

Impatiens personalities are impatient and hectic. They work fast, talk fast, move fast, and even eat fast. The only thing they cannot do quickly is fall asleep, because their busy lifestyle makes them suffer from nervous tension and makes it hard for them to wind down.

Driven by an internal rocket booster, they are always in a rush. They push other people because they have no understanding for people who work more slowly than they do. It drives them mad to watch how other people—in their opinion—waste valuable time. They react angrily and irritably when a project does not progress as quickly as they imagined it. Therefore, they like to work alone, so they do not have to show consideration for others.

In many cases their strong drive for independence causes them to be lonely. If they get sick, they get angry about it and want to be up and about as quickly as possible. They instruct their practitioner to prescribe only fast-acting medication. Because of their hectic work style they tend to be accident prone. Their ability to react instantly prevents the worst.

Impatiens people say about themselves:

- ∾ I am a very impatient person.
- ∾ Nothing can go fast enough for me.
- ∾ I always work fast.
- ∾ My impatience often results in mistakes.
- ∾ I often finish other people's sentences for them.
- ∾ I sometimes take over someone else's job if they act too clumsy. I can't stand watching it.
- ∾ I often urge other people to hurry up.
- ∾ I often say, "Come on, let's go, don't fall asleep, don't act so stupid."
- ∾ When I ask someone to hand me something and he doesn't do it immediately I begin to yell.
- ∾ If I have to wait and I start thinking about what I could have done in the meantime, I become very fidgety.
- ∾ I hate it when I have to wait.
- ∾ When I have to wait somewhere I immediately ask how long it will take and then leave again for a while.
- ∾ If I can't pass a car I sometimes tailgate. It drives me crazy to follow someone who drives slowly.
- ∾ I would rather come a little late than be too early and have to

wait, so I tend to leave the house late and then drive a little faster.

∾ My uncontrollable haste often takes my breath away.

Impatiens people are constantly under inner pressure to do something or to work, because their impatience and petulance represent an inner force that they somehow have to work out. According to their temprament they suffer from inner tension, muscle tightness, back pain, nervous stomach, intestinal problems, nervous twitches, or other symptoms. The increased inner tension often leads to high blood pressure; the fast mental pace often causes an elevated pulse rate.

How does such a high inner speed make it hard for these individuals to cope with a slow-moving environment? On the one hand, it may simply be their temperament; the impetuous and impulsive Aries nature, for example, is well known. On the other hand, there are certain indications that such behavior is influenced by external circumstances such as pregnancy.

Thomas Verny writes in his book *The Spiritual Life of the Newborn* about premature birth: "If childbirth occurs just a few days too early it will be of no consequence. A few weeks are of greater importance, and a premature delivery of a few months can be devastating for the child in a physical and psychological sense. The most harmful effect I observed in my premature patients is that they constantly feel rushed and tortured. This feeling of not being able to catch up or keep up is in my opinion a consequence of a premature birth. They started their life as driven individuals and still feel this way many years later."[3] The birth trauma can therefore play an important role in the creation of negative self images, as we already have seen it in the Rock Rose flower. I will come back to this later in the case of the Star of Bethlehem flower.

Olive *(Olea europaea)*

People who need Olive have in a physical and psychological sense reached the end of their rope. They are exhausted to such an extent that life appears only as a struggle to them. Even day-to-day life activities like washing, brushing one's teeth, or having a bowel movement seem to be insurmountable obstacles. Their faces are pale and expressionless. They seem apathetic and talk only if they are asked something and even then in a low voice. They seem to be without any drive and have only one wish: to sleep.

An Olive state appears after overwork and chronic strain, worries and a long serious illness, in which an all-consuming battle against suffering has been fought. It indicates that all energy reserves have been used up. The affected individuals are—in contrast with Hornbeam—unable to perform their tasks and duties.

People who need Olive say about themselves:

- ∾ I feel so weak, I only want to sleep.
- ∾ My last energy reserves have been spent.
- ∾ I'm so tired that I can hardly walk anymore.
- ∾ I feel so exhausted that I can't enjoy anything.
- ∾ Right now life is just one big weight on my shoulders.
- ∾ I don't want to go on. I am at my wit's end.
- ∾ At work I count the hours until I can go home.

Olive states appear in both moderate and acute forms, such as the ones mentioned above, depending on the depletion and constitution of the individual. An overexertion does not have to be present for a long time. A single event requiring a large amount of strength can be enough to cause later exhaustion. In this case the condition will fade away by itself, because the energy reserves are usually not fully depleted. Olive, however, can hasten the regeneration process.

An Olive state is the result of a prior Impatiens state. Impatiens people almost always live above their energy level because of their overactive lifestyle. Hunger attacks are often an indicator of the depletion of their energy potential. This should signify to them that it's time to face the consequences and lighten up. Otherwise, it can happen that the total exertion of the Olive state can jeopardize the success of their impatiently pursued goals. They often try to overcome the weakness of the Olive state and to continue and complete their work through sheer willpower. This leads to a state of decompensation marked by the Oak flower.

Oak *(Quercus robur)*

Oak types are responsible and reliable people who accomplish many things, but from a false sense of duty they take on many things and sometimes even carry the weight of other people. They never complain and are not disturbed by even the greatest difficulties. When they become ill they want to get better as soon as possible, as do the Impatiens types. They are unhappy with themselves when they have no accomplishments.

Oak people say about themselves:

- ∾ I have a strong sense of duty.
- ∾ I feel responsible for many things and therefore work hard.
- ∾ I demand a lot of myself.
- ∾ I am a virtual workaholic.

- I can't delegate work to others because I feel responsible for it.
- I often stretch my endurance and force myself to go on even when I don't have any strength left. I'll stay at home only with a fever of 104°.
- I keep on working even when I feel unable to do so. Even a headache or faintness can't stop me from working. They'll be gone in a couple of hours anyway. That is the reason why I do not do anything about them.
- I reach my lowest point at around ten thirty at night, but with a second wind I can easily go until one o'clock in the morning.

Oak is the opposite of Gorse. Whereas people who need Gorse are often discouraged and desperate and give up easily, Oak people never lose their faith. They continue working even when they are physically unable and force themselves to do so with enormous willpower. Even in seemingly hopeless situations they continue fighting, if necessary until a complete breakdown.

Vervain people also overwork themselves constantly and tend to step over the point of no return. The difference between the two flowers lies in the motivation, as the following comparison shows.

BEHAVIOR	OAK REASON	VERVAIN REASON
Overwork themselves	Exaggerated sense of duty	Euphoria for the project
Take over the work of others	When they do not get on with it	To show them by any means how to do it, even when it becomes obvious that they are unable to do it themselves

An Oak state is not always easy to recognize, because the individuals are often not aware of what they do to their bodies with their incorrect behavior. On the contrary, they have a good conscience because they believe that they have fulfilled their duty. If the body resists this overexertion through illness, they view it as an obstacle that has to be overcome quickly.

It is usually a clear sign of an Oak state when sick people fight their illnesses with full force, instead of giving in to their bodies' longing for rest and waiting for further developments. An Oak state appears not only after over-work but also after a long-lasting illness or continuing job- or family-related problems, such as an unhappy marriage that must be maintained—for the sake of the children—with extreme effort. The care of a sick relative can also lead to an Oak state.

What leads to these extreme states of physical and psychological tension and stress that make it impossible for the individual to relax?

As we have already seen in the case of Olive, the overactive quality of impatient people easily leads to an energy depletion and consequently to situations of fatigue. The inner impatience and the urge for action often forces these people to go on despite exhaustion and prevents them from resting. They try to get well as soon as possible and force themselves to pull through temporary down phases, because they see rest as a waste of time.

Like Vervain people, they ignore phases of exhaustion over time. Whereas the latter use mainly stimulants like coffee or black tea to eliminate the more mental fatigue, Oak people need a great amount of willpower to overcome their mental and physical exhaustion.

In the long run, an attitude develops that illness and weakness are obstacles to the fulfillment of duties that must be eliminated as soon as possible. This sense of duty serves as an alibi for the exploitation of their health, although they are not necessarily aware of it themselves. If this attitude is not stopped, the individuals hold out until their complete col-lapse. It is often very painful when they finally realize that their real motivation is not their sense of responsibility but an internal holding on to an absolutely overextended lifestyle and work situation, which is com-bined with an inability to let go and relax.

Decompensation flower	Oak
Compensation flower	Olive
Communication flower	Impatiens

Chicory—Red Chestnut—Honeysuckle
❧

Chicory *(Chichorium intybus)*

Chicory types are friendly, helpful people with a deep sense of family. They tenderly care for their relatives, and no work seems too much in this regard. In their helpfulness they often put their own needs last and actually sacrifice themselves for other people. Because they have a strong aversion to solitude, they would like to have the people they love very near to them. Their constant worries about the happiness and well-being of others is no charity at all, however, but rather self-love. They do not help people out of unselfish motives but often demand gratitude. They try to bind other people to them and bring them under their own control. They often claim how much other people owe them to put them under moral pressure.

Chicory people say about themselves:

- ∾ I always think of the well-being of others.
- ∾ I worry about people who are close to me and try to help them.
- ∾ I often make well-intended suggestions for others. If they don't follow them, I involve the whole family if necessary to influence their decision.
- ∾ When my children don't do what I want, I try diplomacy.
- ∾ When I know from the start that my child will resist if I ask him to go shopping with me, I tell him he should stay at home. He then comes without a fuss.
- ∾ Of course I expect something in return when I do someone a big favor.
- ∾ My feelings are easily hurt.
- ∾ I easily feel insulted when someone doesn't do what I want.
- ∾ I'm afraid to be alone.
- ∾ I've lived my life for my son. Now my daughter-in-law has taken him away from me.

Chicory people force their good deeds on others and are easily offended when their help is rejected or their advice is not followed. They feel sorry for themselves and complain, "I only wanted to help you, and now you hurt me so badly. After all that I have done for you? What would you be without me? Where is your gratitude?" They always try to make other people dependent on them or try to dominate an already existing dependency relationship, for example, with children.

They find pleasure in giving advice to other people and like to interfere in affairs that are none of their business. Over time they try to gain more and more influence on the lives of others so they will be asked for advice. If other people, even adult children, make their own decisions without them, they feel grossly offended. They then feel disregarded and resentful for a long time.

Their demand for power is not as obvious as in Vine types, but rather is done in a diplomatic way. Their demands are often so subtle that the other person responds rather willingly, almost as if she perceived herself as being guilty. Their tactic is sometimes so brilliant that in the blink of an eye the other person really believes that what she does is the best.

An old woman who needed nursing home care wanted to be attended only by a certain relative. If she was not available, the old woman would refuse to eat. When the caretaker wanted to go on vacation, she tried to force her to stay home. Her blackmailing went so far that in the end she had to be artificially fed in the hospital.

A student received just enough money from his parents that it was enough for his rent and his general expenses but not enough to buy food, which he received at home. In this way his parents forced him to come home every week although he did not want to. He did not receive the money as a standing money order but as a separate transaction each month. In this way his parents assured that the money would not be taken for granted.

If he did not come home some weekends—despite his financial need—his father would "forget" to send him the money. He then had to call home and thus be reminded of his duties as their child, often in conjunction with the reproachful question whether money was his only connection to his parents. Because he might overdraw his account without a standing money order, he repeatedly had to beg for money when he had extra expenses. His father refused in principle to talk about money on the telephone; therefore, he was forced to make an extra trip home.

A small girl regularly manipulated her playmates by telling them, "If you do not play this game with me, I never will be your friend again."

A patient of mine always had attacks of nausea and restlessness while in my treatment room. In her opinion this was related to some kind of radiation, perhaps from the earth or from electricity. Despite the measurement of a dowser, my treatment room was supposedly polluted with radiation, so I had to do her Bach Flower assessment in the waiting room with a note pad on my lap. My inconvenience—I had to move all my homeopathic materials for the intake interview into the waiting room—did not bother her at all. On the contrary, she gave me the feeling that I had to make some effort for her if I wanted to treat her.

Chicory parents appear to outsiders as good parents, because they care for their children intensively. The fact that these children practically suffocate in their well-guarded home remains hidden, however. The feeling of being closed in and of not getting enough air also expresses itself physically: children of Chicory parents often suffer from asthma. This often creates a vicious circle, because this disease means they need even more care and are therefore more dependent on their parents. Such children usually marry very late—if at all—and often after their mother's death.

The alleged reason that Chicory parents frequently raise their children strictly is that they are responsible for the development of their children and therefore have to act that way to keep their children from harm. In reality it is only a justification for their executive power.

Chicory parents believe that they can get back from their children what they have done for them. This, however, is a mistake, because the affection and love they gave to their children was already given to them in advance by their own parents. In some ways they are "double dipping." For example, a couple complained about the "ingratitude" of their adult son, who moved against their wished to a very distant city: "A mother is not just an outlet to the world. The children also have responsibilities toward their parents."

Chicory people suffer from a variety of illnesses, with which they blackmail those around them for affection. Especially "favored" are those illnesses that draw attention or cause pity. Very good results are produced by heart diseases, because they create fear in others. Illnesses that leave the individual helpless or in need of care almost always create the desired effect. Especially in situations where other people act against their wishes, Chicory people promptly get sick. Some examples are:

- ∾ Their spouse wants a divorce.
- ∾ Their children grow up and leave home.
- ∾ Their spouse wants to start working again.

If Chicory people's hopes are dashed, they might commit suicide under certain circumstances. There are, however, some differences between the Wild Rose and Cherry Plum types:

CHICORY TYPES	WILD ROSE TYPES	CHERRY PLUM TYPES
Try suicide because they cannot achieve what they want	Want to die because everything appears to be meaningless	Break down because they cannot withstand the inner pressure
Motive: extortion	Motive: resignation	Motive: a rash act
Have made previous suicide threats	Make suicidal tendencies known only to close friends	Wail to others that they will go crazy, but this is not usually taken seriously
The suicide attempt committed when external circumstances seem favorable	Suicide is planned over a long period	Suicide happens completely unexpected
The suicide is planned to happen at the right time	The suicide is planned to be successful	The suicide is not planned

The Chicory state is hard to diagnose in adults because they are usually unaware of their state of mind. They often justify their demands on their children with the biblical law, "Honor thy mother and father." The significant tip is usually given by the relatives, provided they are aware of their oppression. Chicory children on the other hand are easily recognized by their merciless wailing when they are denied something. They often try to drum up sympathy; this is especially successful in the case of parents who lack willpower and therefore easily let themselves be tyrannized.

A clear indication of a Chicory state is the extreme fear of being alone. Therapy-resistant illnesses of any kind also indicate Chicory, because the patients might gain from their ailments and do not actually wish to get well. In the case of hysterical symptoms one should think about Chicory, because these are also designed to attract attention.

The Chicory portrait is best characterized as an escape from oneself into another person. One's own identity is thereby projected onto another person. Chicory people make other people dependent on them because they themselves are dependent; without others their own life seems meaningless.

The Chicory person turns toward his own personality and finally toward his own self through the internal process of separation from his surroundings is not accomplished without therapeutic help (with or without Bach Flowers). The solution for the conflict must come from his environment. Götz Blome writes: "It is extremely harmful to go along with the Chicory patient's fears (and then pat oneself on the back for helping). He must be liberated from exactly this pathological emotional dependency and the constant desire to receive attention. If such a relationship already exists, the process will not occur without crises—mostly of a healing nature."[4]

Red Chestnut *(Aesculus carnea)*

Red Chestnut people live in constant fear and worry about other people. It seems that their thoughts are solely occupied with the well-being and health of the other members of their family, friends, and acquaintances. They often foresee problems and imagine worst-case scenarios. They suspect a serious disease in their relatives' minor ailments and malaise. When a family member does not come home on time, they fear the worst. Red Chestnut parents are scared to death when their children go away on a class trip for several days. They demand that their children call every night to make sure that nothing bad has happened to them. Out of worry they constantly want to know where their relatives are.

Red Chestnut people say about themselves:

    ∾ I worry constantly about other people.

     ✿ I always live in fear that something might happen to my
       children, that they might have to suffer.

     ✿ I'm always afraid that something bad might happen to
       someone in my family.

     ✿ I worry not only about my family but also about my friends.

     ✿ I often wish I could take on the pain of my children.

     ✿ If someone in my family takes a drive, he has to call when he
       has arrived, otherwise I start worrying.

     ✿ When I send my daughter to school I'm afraid that I'll receive
       the news that something terrible has happened to her.

Red Chestnut is the decompensation flower for Chicory. A Red Chestnut state is the justification for the power demanded in the Chicory state. In this way the accusations of patronization and oppression and the possible evolution of self doubt are pushed aside. They have already justified their behavior in the Chicory state with the statement that they act in the interest of others only because they worry about their well-being. In the Red Chestnut state this subconscious excuse leads to a situation in which they really do worry.

The escape from themselves has taken the form of self-alienation. Where before they indirectly ruled over other people through their diplomatic behavior, they are now indirectly ruled by others because their thoughts focus only on the welfare of these people. Because thier own fears and worries are projected onto others, they lose their self-awareness. The escape from themselves has therefore been successful; but at what price?

Their deep inner conflict is not obvious to the outside insofar as their selfless Samaritan-like care is considered a noble character trait. For instance, a religious education combined with the Christian ideal of charity may lead to the false conclusion that they do not really love other people unless they worry about them. The moral superiority of these people is just an excuse, however, because the motivation is wrong. The better way to help people would be to entrust them to God's care instead of worrying about their fate. A lack of faith in God and love that is not genuine leads to this perverted form of human care.

The fears and worries of Red Chestnut people are of no real help to others. On the contrary, they are a restrictive burden. The mental vibration of fear transfers to the people at whom they are directed. Their effect is absolutely tangible for sensitive people. It is known of Edward Bach that every thought of depression, worry, or fear for another person caused him acute pain.[5] The damage caused by excessive worrying can also be material: Red Chestnut people often tend to immediately give their children strong medication for minor ailments, for example, because they fear that a serious disease could develop. Because they only want to prevent the worst, they do not realize that the constant suppression of minor complaints and the frequent ingestion of strong medications can be harmful to the child's organism.

Red Chestnut, as we have already noticed, shares some characteristics with Chicory. In some cases the flowers cannot easily be distinguished from each other, because the boundaries between the two states are fluid.

Honeysuckle *(Lonicera caprifolium)*

Honeysuckle people live more in the past than in the present. Because the latter does not have much to offer them, they escape into their memories of better times. They put all present things in relation to the past and feel that everything in the past was better than today. Their unsatisfying present situation adds glory to the past. This leads to the belief that they cannot expect any further happiness. In talking to others they always end up on the "good old days" and often start their sentences with the comment, "Those were the days when . . . " In their daydreams they hang on to their favorite memories. They lack concentration at work because their thoughts drift away.

Honeysuckle people say about themselves:

- ᔑ The best time of my life was the past. I always think about it; I can remember exactly my thoughts and even smells.
- ᔑ I live in my memories, especially those of my childhood.
- ᔑ I often think about my childhood and wistfully wish for it to come back.
- ᔑ I often revel in my nostalgic feelings.
- ᔑ I often feel homesick.
- ᔑ I often dream of the "good old days."
- ᔑ I often wistfully think back on the time when we were children.
- ᔑ I often long for the time of my childhood.

Honeysuckle states often occur in the following situations:

- ᔑ After a move
- ᔑ After the loss of a loved one
- ᔑ When the children are grown up and move out of the house
- ᔑ After a separation from a spouse that is later regretted
- ᔑ After retirement
- ᔑ On the deathbed

After her only son moved out of the house, one patient placed the little toy duck of her daughter, dead for twenty-five years, at eye level in the kitchen, just to be reminded of the good old times. Her motivation was the desperate longing for the presence of her daughter. If only her daughter were alive, she would not be alone now.

Another patient of mine told me of a yearning she had had for a long time but could not pinpoint. It was simply a wistful feeling and a strong longing for something about which she did not really know. After reincarnation therapy she told me that she had remembered an experience from a former life that was the reason for her longing. She now knew what she was yearning for. This undefined wistful feeling always reappeared in situations similar to those in the "past." After treatment with Honeysuckle, both the yearning and the accompanying physical ailments quickly disappeared.

Honeysuckle people refer in principle to an actually experienced situation. Otherwise Clematis would be the right flower. Honeysuckle patients often suffer from heart ailments; they try to remind themselves symbolically to bring their "heart," that is, their feelings, back from the past to the present time. A Honeysuckle state is a decompensation state, although the symptoms do not look that dramatic at first glance. These individuals live with their thoughts and feelings in the past while their bodies are in the present. As a result of this split they use only a tiny fraction of their intellectual potential. The escape from the self has entered the last phase, the escape from the present. The self-alienation of the Red Chestnut state has led to a state that can best characterized with the expression "out of touch with reality."

The individuals do not find their way in the present time because their mind remains in the past. Their perspective is always backwards-looking, because the future does not offer any hope. They are emotionally frozen and live like shadows that are there but do not participate in life.

Decompensation flower	Honeysuckle
Compensation flower	Red Chestnut
Communication flower	Chicory

MIMULUS——HEATHER——MUSTARD

Mimulus (*Mimulus guttatus*)

Mimulus people are anxious, extremely sensitive, and most of all frightened. They seem to be in every sense of the word living mimosas. The list of things they are oversensitive to is long, and it is sometimes hard for people around them to respect their fears. They are sensitive to:

- ✑ Loud noises
- ✑ Loud talking
- ✑ Bright light
- ✑ Neon light
- ✑ Unfriendly words
- ✑ Cold
- ✑ Conflict
- ✑ Other people's aggression

The prominent feature of Mimulus people is their fear, which in contrast to Aspen people focuses on real objects. Most often these are everyday items such as:

- ✑ Illnesses
- ✑ Storms
- ✑ Water
- ✑ Pain
- ✑ Shots
- ✑ The dentist
- ✑ Accidents
- ✑ Driving
- ✑ Flying
- ✑ Burglars
- ✑ Animals, e.g., dogs

Mimulus people say about themselves:

- ✑ Driving used to be no problem for me, but now I'm afraid that something might happen to me.
- ✑ It's terrible. My fear of all kinds of things prevents me from doing the things I actually should do.
- ✑ No one can convince me to fly in an airplane. I would really like to do it, but my fear of crashing is too great.
- ✑ I become very frightened in high places, for example, standing on a ladder or climbing a tree.
- ✑ If I look out the window from the second floor I become panicky. I go out on the balcony only with mixed feelings.
- ✑ I'm constantly afraid of losing my job. Every time I'm called by my boss, I'm afraid he will give me my notice.

Their sensitive constitution makes life hard for Mimulus people. Without intending to, they often tyrannize people by forcing them to respect their extreme sensitivities and fears.

One somewhat exaggerated example will portray how this takes place in daily life. Assume a Mimulus person gets invited to stay overnight at his host's house. Because the apartment is very small, he sleeps with his host in the same bedroom. This may lead to a well-known ritual for the Mimulus person: The host must go to bed before the sensitive guest, because he would not be able to fall asleep at a different time than he is used to. The shutters must be half open because the guest is afraid of the dark. The alarm clock has to be removed from the bedroom because the ticking noise makes it hard for him to go to sleep. The big grandfather clock in the living room has to be stopped because the stroke of the clock would probably scare him in his sleep. During the first half of the night the host is awakened several times and asked to stop snoring. Finally, in the middle of the night the host is awakened again by a completely agitated guest with the urgent plea for his own room, because he has not been able to close his eyes for one second. The host politely leaves the bedroom and sleeps on the living room couch.

The next morning the coffee has to be poured out. The host forgot that it makes his guest nervous. Fortunately, there is some milk left in the refrigerator. The usual music accompanying breakfast also cannot be turned on because it also makes his guest nervous. The visit to the museum is cut short because the museum is rather crowded, and the guest is afraid of crowds. The visit to the radio tower turns out to be rather difficult because they climb the steps to avoid the elevator. It is not easy to find the right restaurant now because one is too loud and the other is too smoky. The plan to go dancing also turns out to be a failure because the music is too loud and the bright light of the light show is unbearable for the guest. Finally, they agree to go to the movies. The movie is not very entertaining, but on the other hand the theater is almost empty.

Even if this example is exaggerated, it portrays Mimulus people quite well; they manage their existence in this way and are almost unable to survive in an insensitive environment. Their lives appear almost like a caricature to others; however, it is their reality.

The less they look after themselves, the more sensitive they will be. The "freedom" of a good strong cup of coffee comes back to haunt them just like a boomerang the following night. It is almost impossible for them to break this vicious cycle. Under the guidance of a therapist, Mimulus people can help themselves live a worthy life again. As a result of the imminent danger of falling back into the same patterns, which are ingrained in the psyche like computer programs, external help is needed for a case as extreme as that mentioned above.

Anticipation anxieties, as described in the literature, are also part of the Mimulus flower. Larch people also suffer from them. Different motives make it possible to distinguish the flowers from each other quite well.

MINIMULUS	LARCH
Anxiety about new situations; for example, the first day of school	Anticipation anxiety; for example, fear of something new, fear of failure, fear of embarrassment
Fear related to an object, such as a stranger	Fear related to the self; subjective fear
Examination anxiety—fear of the examiner	Examination anxiety—fear of failure
Cause: anxious nature	Cause: lack of self-esteem

Mimulus people often need the base flower Larch, so that in treatment both flowers are often given together.

Mimulus people are often reserved and try to hide their fears from those around them. In this way they often go unnoticed, but their extreme sensitivity does not stay hidden. Starting in the state of compensation, when their suffering becomes so overwhelming that they start to cling to other people, it becomes obvious that deep inner problems lurk behind the now-apparent behavior.

Heather *(Calluna vulgaris)*

Heather people always need an audience. They tell everyone who comes along what is on their mind at the moment. They believe that those around them have an interest in hearing about their latest exciting experience. They do not keep secrets and even talk to strangers about their problems. The main thing is to have someone who listens to them. They like to interfere in other people's conversation because they feel approached by everyone who stands close to them. They take over the conversation with their non-stop talking and hardly let anyone else talk. At the same time, in their aggressiveness they move closer and closer to their victims, who then cannot withdraw. The actions of Heather people can be explained in short by the idiom: "He came, saw—and talked!"[6]

Heather people say about themselves:

- ∞ I need a lot of love and affection. If I have problems I need to talk with someone about them.
- ∞ I often suffer under conditions where I feel really bad. In such situations I need someone to talk to.
- ∞ I quickly feel lonely when I am all alone. I then have to talk to someone on the phone, and it doesn't matter who is on the other end.
- ∞ I often cling to other people; I have a very needy nature.
- ∞ I often feel pity for myself.
- ∞ When I'm sick, my husband is not allowed to leave my bedside.
- ∞ My doctor told me not to concentrate too much on physical symptoms, because my illness is pure imagination.
- ∞ My friends complain that I always talk but never listen.
- ∞ I can't attend any gathering at which I am not allowed to talk.
- ∞ I put up with a lot to be the center of attention.
- ∞ I won't stop until everything in my club centers around me.
- ∞ I change clothes three or four times a day until I feel certain I will attract the attention of other people.
- ∞ If I met a rich man who could offer me everything and who could make me famous, I would marry him at once.

Heather people are completely self centered and in their thoughts completely preoccupied with themselves. For this reason it is hard for them to listen, especially because they have no interest in other people's problems. Everything is centered around their own personality. Their sentences therefore mostly start with "I." As a result of their inability to be alone they virtually cling to other people. Edward Bach characterizes them as "burrs." They command from others the affection they require to satisfy their extreme need for sympathy. They are not aware that other people find their behavior taxing and soon listen to them only to be polite.

Many times Heather patients will tell the whole history of their illness in the waiting room. When they finally have arrived at their therapist, they start pouring their hearts out. In their hypochondriacal behavior they observe themselves very closely and want to show off all their symptoms. Under these circumstances they blow things out of proportion and make a mountain out of a molehill. They pity themselves and desire the same pity from their counterparts.

Heather children can be recognized by their interference in the conversation of adults and by their not letting the conversation continue. They try every-thing to get attention and to be the center of attention. When they do not succeed through normal behavior they start to act silly and play the fool. Often they even put up with punishment for their undisciplined behavior, because this kind of affection is still better than no affection for them.

Here are two examples: In my office, an eight-year-old boy always tried to disturb my conversation with his mother by whistling. After she told him to stop he started with other noises, such as loud smacking or clicking his tongue. His mother told me that in school he tried to be the worst student to attract attention. His goals were to be the laziest, naughtiest, and meanest child of all. In this way he was frequently able to be the center of attention.

A young lady suddenly started screaming at a party: "For God's sake—this child is drunk!" Everyone looked at a little three-year-old boy who was staggering through the room and who obviously had problems walking straight without falling down. He stumbled through the room past the guests as if in a parade, in which everyone held their breath. Some people were shocked, and others thought it was funny. After a while the boy suddenly walked normally again; the show was over and he had achieved what he wanted. He had not taken one sip of alcohol.

A Heather state is the consequence of a previous Mimulus state. Whereas during the Mimulus state the individuals do not talk about their fears and problems, they now fall into the compensatory Heather state. Because their fears and consequent suffering has become unbearable for their sensitive natures, they move to the other extreme and talk about them with everyone. The lesson that should have been learned during the Mimulus state, namely, to develop virtues like courage and self-esteem, should have been the basis for the positive attributes of the Heather flower, empathy and helpfulness. This was not successful, so the individuals are completely dependent on the helpfulness of other people. The Heather person's misconception is that she must look in other people for something she can find only in the depth of her own soul, namely, the trust that overcomes fear.

Mustard *(Sinapis arvensis)*

Individuals who need Mustard suffer from periods of deep depression, which appear without any apparent reason or incident and disappear as suddenly as they come on. A cold, dark cloud seems to overshadow them. They describe this state as a feeling of total inner emptiness, in which everything seems to be senseless and dark, as if someone has turned out the light. These episodes, which occur suddenly like lightning out of a clear blue sky, range from melancholy, sadness, lack of motivation, and unexplainable bad moods to deep depression.

People who need Mustard say about themselves:

- ∾ My mood is often as cloudy as the weather. I don't know why.
- ∾ Off and on I suffer from unexplainable sadness.
- ∾ I frequently suffer from depression that comes on without any reason.
- ∾ Sometimes a deep sadness and melancholy suddenly take hold of me.
- ∾ I have a good husband, two nice children, a house, and a nice piece of land; I really don't know where this depression comes from.
- ∾ I sometimes feel locked in a bell jar from which I can't escape.

Mustard people often appear to be introverted and slowed in their physical reactions. They are often virtually paralyzed by their melancholy. In their desire to be left alone with their problems they often withdraw from their environment. They often suffer from a lack of appetite, sleep disturbances, headaches and other indefinable physical symptoms. These complaints do not necessarily occur in every Mustard patient; in mild cases only an unfounded melancholy without any concomitant symptoms may be present. They should be seen as indications of Mustard, especially when the cause of the complaints is not known.

For this reason Götz Blome also recommends Mustard for so-called latent depression, which is hidden and subconscious to the patient and which accounts for physical ailments with no organic cause. He writes: "In latent depression Mustard is recommended. It is possible to recognize the depressive component in concomitant physical symptoms . . . through a close study of the whole person. In principle, the organism always tries to divert insoluble emotional problems into the body or to make them conscious."[7] It should be mentioned, though, that the diagnosis "latent depression" is often mistakenly made, because in many cases a cause of illness can be found through natural methods.

Contrary to Mustard, an external cause for the depression can be found in the Gentian depression. It is therefore defined as exogenous (coming from the outside) and reactive (through stimuli from the environment).

A Mustard state is the result of a prior Heather state. Heather people look in others for what they cannot find in the depth of their own soul: trust that can overpower the Mimulus state. Because the outside world cannot offer them this primal trust, in the state of decompensation they will sense that they are missing something, but they do not know what it is. Contact to their own higher self is blocked, and it is therefore impossible for them to find strength in themselves. This leads to a feeling of inner emptiness, which appears to have no reason because they are not conscious of this feeling of emptiness.

Decompensation flower	Mustard
Compensation flower	Heather
Communication flower	Mimulus

CLEMATIS——IMPATIENS——MUSTARD

Clematis *(Clematis vitalba)*

Clematis people are daydreamers. Many times they are absentminded; they dream with their eyes open and live more in their dream world than in reality. They show minimal interest in daily affairs and escape from harsh reality into a dream world, in which everything seems more beautiful and harmonious. To those around them they appear to be inattentive and uninterested. They often seem to be tired, and one gets the feeling that they are not completely there. This becomes visible through small accidents, for example, when they trip, fall down, get caught on something, bump into other people, or drop things. Especially in children one can observe this behavior quite frequently.

Because their thoughts constantly wander, they lack concentration at work and easily become distracted. Most of all, they are extremely forgetful, which is based on their general lack of interest in external affairs. Their fantasy world keeps them occupied to such a degree that it is hard for them to manage real life.

Once they become sick, they undertake hardly any efforts to get better; on the contrary, they often give the impression that they use their illness as an escape from reality. To lie in bed and float in their dreams seems to be more attractive to them than real life. They tend to sleep a great deal anyway, because they do not think that they would miss out on anything. They prefer to withdraw from society and to be left alone with their thoughts.

Clematis people say about themselves:

- I am often deep in thoughts—usually not about real things but about fantasies and dreams.
- I am often not aware of what goes on around me.
- I perform many things in a trancelike state, because I'm constantly dreaming. These dreams are often about things I'd like to have but can't.
- I have many fantasies about the future.

- ॐ I always dream about making the world a better place.
- ॐ Even when I have company I pursue my thoughts and often don't notice what happens around me. When someone asks me a question I often get startled.
- ॐ When we visit friends my husband always scolds me afterward because I never listen to the conversation but rather let my thoughts wander.
- ॐ When I watch TV I often don't follow the show at all, because my thoughts are somewhere else.
- ॐ I often get lost when I drive because I don't pay much attention to where I'm going.
- ॐ Before I start work I often just dream along for a while, so that many projects remain unfinished. I then have to hurry to get things done.
- ॐ I slowly become desperate because my work doesn't seem to progress, mainly because I drift off in my thoughts and start daydreaming.
- ॐ Once when I was preoccupied, I first carried the milk down to the basement, then into my bedroom, until I finally became aware of what I actually wanted to do. Only then did I bring it to the kitchen.
- ॐ I often forget appointments. That's why everyone gives me calendars as presents.

Honeysuckle, White Chestnut, and Chestnut Bud people all show excessive mental activity. The differences, however, exist in the kinds of thoughts that occupy each type. A comparison of the flower remedies will illustrate this:

CLEMATIS	HONEYSUCKLE	WHITE CHESTNUT	CHESTNUT BUD
Fantasies, daydreams, wishful thinking	Nostalgia, longing for the good old days	Irritating thoughts that one can't "shut off"	Plans, ideas always two steps ahead in one's mind
Thoughts about the future	Thoughts about the past	Compulsive thoughts, constant inner dialogue	Thoughts about what to do next

The lack of drive, one of the main symptoms of Clematis, also appears in Wild Rose, Hornbeam and Olive. The conditions that lead to the symptoms are completely different, however, as the following comparison will show.

CLEMATIS	WILD ROSE	HORNBEAM	OLIVE	MUSTARD
Live more in a fantasy world with no interest in the present	Inner resignation; inner capitulation; nothing has any meaning	Mentally strained, exhausted, want to sleep all the time	Total exhaustion; unable to perform any physical labor	Without any drive in depressive phases
Chronic state	Length depends on external circumstances	Mostly acute; sometimes can turn into a chronic state	Acute state	Temporary state

Clematis people often suffer from visual or auditory disturbances. The body tries to express in this way its lack of interest in the external world. Circulation problems, cold hands and feet, and a pale skin color also indicate that the individuals do not participate in life in an active way. On the contrary, the Clematis state has a certain affinity to death, because life has no special meaning for them.

The Clematis flower counteracts the tendency of the mind to drift away and therefore can be a great help in some cases of unconsciousness, coma, or collapse. It helps to restore consciousness to the body and can therefore offer help in emergency situations, and under certain circumstances can save lives. For this reason it is the main ingredient of the Rescue Remedy (see chapter 6, "Rescue Remedy").

Impatiens *(Impatiens glandulifera)*

The Impatiens state originates out of the Clematis state as a form of compensation. The effects of this state are no different from the ones already described in the Impatiens state of the track Impatiens—Olive—Oak. The only difference in this case is that the individuals do not react impatiently by nature. They develop this behavior as the result of their constant mental absence and their flight into the fantasy world while in the Clematis state. Clematis people often startle suddenly from their daydreams by looking at a clock. They become painfully aware that they waste a lot of time through their mental digression and are now forced to catch up with everything they have missed in their absentmindedness. Through this necessary rush they are quickly brought back to reality, from which they can escape again only after they have done their duties. Because of this self-induced stress, they often act excessively and try impatiently to finish their work as soon as possible to end their trip to reality. In this way from a passive, introverted yin state the hyperactive, extroverted yang state emerges, represented by the Impatiens flower.

Mustard *(Sinapis arvensis)*

Resulting from the urge to catch up with what was neglected while daydreaming, in order to return again to daydreaming, a state of decompensation has emerged. This leads to a hectic way of working, which makes life more difficult for the individual and, therefore, makes it seem to be even more of a burden. The difference between harsh reality and the safe world of dreams becomes even more extreme. In the reality of daily life a vague and undefined feeling of loss emerges over time. The less time that remains for dreaming or the less it it is possible to make the dreams come true, the more this feeling increases in intensity.

The sensation that something is missing, but not knowing what it might be, leads in the state of decompensation to the feeling of emptiness, as already described in the track Mimulus—Heather—Mustard. Times of melancholy and depression bring this inner vacuum to the surface of the consciousness and signal that the entrance to the source of real happiness in the depth of their own soul is buried.

Decompensation flower	Mustard
Compensation flower	Impatiens
Communication flower	Clematis

4

LARCH:
THE FOUNDATION FLOWER

Larch *(Larix decidua)* people perceive themselves as less capable than other people. Because of their lack of self-esteem, they doubt their own abilities and admire other people's success. They are constantly tormented by the fear of failing. When greatly challenged or tested they often lose courage and give up early. Some are so convinced of their incompetence that they don't even try many things. They are therefore perceived as cowardly.

They feel inferior to other people, and their fear of making a fool of themselves makes them shy and inhibited. As a result of their inferiority complex they pay great respect to authority figures and willingly subordinate themselves. They are sensitive to critique and disapproval and react intensely when hurt, often losing their temper.

People who need Larch say about themselves:

- ∾ I doubt whether I can live up to my own expectations.
- ∾ I have little self-esteem. I'm often surprised when I'm successful.
- ∾ I don't believe in myself.
- ∾ I feel afraid of failure.
- ∾ I don't often dare to approach a woman.
- ∾ I suffer from anxiety.
- ∾ I'm afraid of everything new in my life.
- ∾ When I drive to an unfamiliar place I often become insecure and afraid that I won't be able to find my way around.
- ∾ I suffer from examination anxiety weeks before the test.
- ∾ I feel insecure among other people, because I speak English with an accent.

∾ I gave up on sports when I was a child because I'm so clumsy.

∾ If I'm not able to achieve something I feel like a complete failure.

∾ I sometimes feel inferior.

∾ I suffer from impotence.

∾ I'm sensitive about criticism and disapproval.

Larch children are shy, blush easily, and out of nervousness are often unable to talk. The reason for stuttering (if not induced through a shock experience) lies often in a Larch state.

Larch also functions as the main remedy for impotence. Even if self-esteem has not been affected by this problem and did not play a role in its development, it will sooner or later be lost, because most people are programmed by society to identify male potency with vigor and strength. Everyone who fails in bed is generally seen as a failure per se.

In some ways Larch has certain similarities to other flowers. But it is easily distinguished from them, as the comparison on the following page shows.

Larch states are deeply rooted in the personality structure. They can also occur through external influences, however, especially during childhood, when the affirmation of the self through its surroundings is still missing, or when the child may get programmed in a negative way. The remark "You can't do that—you're too young" becomes second nature to children if they hear it often enough. In certain situations they react accordingly from the start and will not even try certain things. The statement "I can't do it" has deeply imprinted itself like a mantra in their minds.

Remarks like, "You silly one," which are not meant by the parent to do harm, can also leave scars in children. Everything they hear from older and more "experienced" people they accept as the truth without questioning. The impression forms unconsciously; the individual feels intellectually inferior. A patient once told me that during childhood his mother told him he had two left hands. This was completely unjustified; meanwhile, he turned out to be very talented in crafts. The mother compared him with his father, who as an adult was certainly more skilled.

We cannot apply our own standards to our children but instead have to adjust to the child's standards. Self-esteem should be reinforced and built on. Rather than reproaching we should get used to motivating them in a positive way. The statement, "Not bad for a beginner, but if you practice more, you will be able to do it even better" sounds much more encouraging to children's ears than a devastating critique.

LARCH	GENTIAN	CERATO	ELM
Question success because they do not believe they could do it.	Are afraid that something will go wrong		
Have doubts about what they *can* do.		Do not know what they *should* do.	
Expect failure, because they doubt their capabilities.	Expect failure because of unfortunate circumstances.		
Suffer from examination anxiety, which starts weeks before the test and creases continuously the closer the date. The anxiety expresses itself as despair—they would rather quit before they actually start.			Suffer from examination anxiety, which begins during the test or suddenly appears shortly before, completely unexpectedly. The anxiety expresses itself as "black out" during the test: the learned material is suddenly gone.
Cause: lack of self-esteem.	Cause: pessimistic attitude.	Cause: do not trust their own opinion.	Cause: expecta-expectations are too high.

I classify Larch as the foundation flower because many emotional disturbances are based on a lack of self-esteem. It cannot be related to only one specific track, but can be combined with each of them. The application is determined by the indication. The biggest effect, however, is achieved in combination with communication flowers, because it will enhance their effect.

LARCH	HOLLY	WILLOW
Admire other people for their success	Envy other people for their success	Embittered about their own failures

Here is one example to illustrate this:

- ✢ Given alone, Larch strengthens self-esteem.
- ✢ Larch in combination with Pine also strengthens self-esteem, while Pine eases feelings of guilt.
- ✢ Larch, given in combination with Centaury, can help individuals build up their willpower after having regained their self-esteem. The effect of Centaury will occur more rapidly through the combination with Larch than as a single application.

Larch as a foundation flower is used especially in combinations with strong yin-oriented communication flowers like Agrimony, Centaury, Cerato, Gentian, and Mimulus.

5

OUTER FLOWERS

Star of Bethlehem *(Ornithologalum umbellatum)*

Star of Bethlehem is the remedy for unresolved situations:

- Emotional shock
- Deep grief
- Emotional despair
- After disappointments
- After accidents or disasters
- After the loss of a family member
- After bad news
- Against the effect of a shock dating far back in the past, for example, shock during childhood, birth trauma, and pregnancy

Physical injuries also indicate Star of Bethlehem, because they represent a shock experience for the afflicted body cells, for example:

- Concussion
- Skull fracture
- Spinal injuries
- Fractures, and so forth

Star of Bethlehem people have been injured, which has made them vulnerable. The shock has left behind a deep emotional wound. With every trauma that opens up the old wound, the existing pain becomes deeper and their level of tolerance decreases, so that after a while even minor events upset them. In extreme cases this can even lead to hysterical reactions.

People who need Star of Bethlehem report:

- ∿ I have been deeply disappointed.
- ∿ For days I can't forget unpleasant events.
- ∿ Unpleasant past events reappear in my memory over and over again, sometimes in the form of dreams.
- ∿ When I think about the past I often have to cry.
- ∿ As a child I saw an accident that still haunts me today.
- ∿ Once a drunk person ran into my car. This was a bad shock and still disturbs me sometimes.
- ∿ Since my uncle died I feel an inner void that will never again be filled.
- ∿ My mother spanked me a lot. To this day I haven't been able to forget this.

An emotional shock causes a convulsion of the whole energetic system. If not processed, this misinformation in the energetic system will lead to dysfunction of all kinds. For this reason the Star of Bethlehem state can be seen as a kind of block in therapy. It does not matter how long ago the shock occurred. Long-forgotten childhood shocks, the birth trauma, and even emotional trauma during the mother's pregnancy can result in a range of disorders that become apparent only in a later stage of life.

Thomas Verny writes:

Birth . . . is the first physical and psychological experience of shock that a child has to go through, and it will never entirely forget it. It experiences moments of incredible sensual bliss—moments in which every inch of its body is surrounded by the mother's warm fluids and massaged by her muscles. These moments, however, are alternately replaced by others charged with pain and fear. . . .

One moment the child is swimming joyfully in a lake of warm amniotic fluid, in the next one it is pushed into the birth canal, where it undergoes a great ordeal lasting many hours. Most horrible are the mother's contractions, which come down on it with the force of an anvil. . . .

How these immense forces of contraction feel we can only imagine. Recently conducted radiological tests, however, show that with every contraction the baby is swinging its arms and legs wildly, as if writhing in pain.[1]

Dr. Verny's observations are confirmed by subjective experiences in the form of memories of the birth, which can be triggered through the use of regression techniques such as rebirthing, reincarnation therapy, and hypnosis. Often the postdelivery experiences were traumatic, for example, the feeling of expulsion; the separation from the mother; the cold, bright room; being touched by unknown people; the feeling of helplessness.

Thorwald Dethlefsen writes about traumas during pregnancy: "Compared with the prenatal experiences, the childhood experiences of the first years of life are harmless episodes."[2] The fetus is completely aware of the mother's experiences. It shares her feelings and experiences her fears, sorrows, pain, and most of all her feelings toward itself: happiness about the developing life or her (often unconscious) resentment against the child, and likewise any unsuccessful attempts at abortion.

The following example shows to what extent the experiences during pregnancy still live on in later life: "As a young man I was stunned by my unusual ability to play some musical compositions without the score. Once, while conducting a piece, I suddenly became aware of the cello line and knew how the music would go on without turning the page. One day I mentioned this to my mother, who is a professional cellist. I thought it would also surprise her that it was the the the cello line that stood out so clearly for me. She was also stunned; however, when I told her the specific pieces, the riddle solved itself. All the compositions that I remembered without knowing the written scores were the ones she had played while she was pregnant with me."[3]

I experienced a similar phenomenon after the birth of my son. When I sang the song my wife had sung almost every day during her pregnancy, he would instantly quiet down. If I sang a different but similar-sounding song, though, he would immediately start to cry again.

Trauma surrounding conception, for example, rape, will influence later life and show itself in the future sexual behavior of the individual.

Under certain circumstances Rock Rose can be used for traumatic external influences. The comparison on the following page will give a better idea of the differences between the two flowers. In acute fright and shock situations Rescue Remedy is usually given, a ready-made mixture for all kinds of emergency, which contains both flowers.

In all therapy-resistant illnesses one has to consider Star of Bethlehem, because in these cases a possible emotional trauma might be the cause of the complaints. Psychosomatic complaints in particular are often caused by trauma that is unknown to the individuals because they have displaced it from their memory: neurosis, hysterical symptoms, thyroid problems, dysphagia, functional heart disease, bronchial asthma, sexual dysfunction, and nervous bladder. Because everyone will have an emotional shock some time in life, therapists in principle will add Star of Bethlehem to the first Bach flower remedy, thus eliminating trauma-related therapy blocks from the start.

STAR OF BETHLEHEM	ROCK ROSE
Psychological shock	Panic, mortal fear
Example: One witnesses an accident and sees a badly injured, bleeding accident victim.	Example: one is involved in an accident and is paralyzed by fear. One barely escapes death.
Extreme yin state	Extreme yang state
The acute shock symtoms show a certain resemblance to that of the homeopathic remedy Opium.	The acute anxiety symptoms show a certain resemblance to that of the homeopathic remedy Aconitum.
Effects: The energetic system is blocked; over time consequential damage will occur.	Effects: The fear is displaced. This leads to a compensatory Agrimony state. Consequential damages will become visible only in the state of decompensation.

Elm *(Ulmus procera)*

An acute Elm state occurs in situations in which too much is expected from the individuals at the moment. They feel overwhelmed and incapable of meeting the task. These are usually capable and efficient people, who usually finish their tasks without any great difficulties. Their work at the moment, however, has exceeded their capabilities. The reason for the excess strain can be higher environmental expectations (for example, examinations, promotions, situations that require a great deal of responsibility, time pressure through deadlines, being left completely alone) as well as too high expectations of themselves (Vervain type).

People who need the Elm flower say about themselves:

- I feel right now that I can't live up to my expectations.
- I took on more than I could handle. I can't possibly do all of this.
- I'm afraid that I won't be able to manage all this work.
- I feel absolutely burned out and unable to finish the work assigned to me. I have so many things to do that I don't know where to start.
- My new project doesn't let me rest. I'm afraid this is too

much for me. I'm always thinking about what I have to do. This makes me nervous and doesn't let me sleep.

∾ My work looks like an insurmountable obstacle.

∾ I often have blackouts in school. Suddenly I can't concentrate anymore.

∾ Many times during a test I suddenly feel afraid, become insecure, and do not remember anything. I actually feel capable and am not afraid of the test; but as soon as I'm asked something, everything I know disappears.

∾ In my job interview I suddenly lost all courage and was unable to say a word.

∾ When I have to substitute unexpectedly, I can't adjust to the changed situation fast enough and feel overwhelmed. I'm not very good at taking over the class of another teacher. I often stand in front of the class and don't know what to do. It feels like everything I learned during my training is suddenly gone.

∾ In the game I suddenly have a blackout and perform much worse than during practice. It always starts shortly before the match, when I see the opponent and I suddenly become aware of the expectations that are laid on me. Once I put a Walkman on shortly before the game and walked around outside to distract myself. Then I performed extremely well.

People who need Elm lose their self-esteem only for a short time as a result of excessive demands, whereas Larch people doubt their abilities almost all the time. The periods of weakness appear in Elm, in contrast to Olive and Hornbeam, only in conjunction with excessive demands and not feeling up to the situation. They appear more unexpectedly and dramatically and can lead in extreme cases to a nervous breakdown. Elm states in general are characterized by the sudden breakdown of psychological and sometimes physical strength. These accompanying symptoms can appear:

∾ Difficulties swallowing
∾ Lack of concentration
∾ Extreme nervousness
∾ Circulation problems
∾ Heart palpitations
∾ Nervous breakdown
∾ Fainting spells

Walnut *(Juglans regia)*

Walnut is a flower for a new beginning. It helps people with great changes in their lives to adapt to the new life circumstances, to let go of the old and to accept the new. It is also called the "breakthrough flower." It is the remedy that helps us come through all periods of change without regret, without looking back at the past, without fears for the future, and therefore spares us the intellectual and physical strain that is usually connected with such events."

Walnut is also helpful in phases of inner change, hormonal adaptation, and intellectual development. The typical areas for application are:

- ∾ Moving
- ∾ Career change
- ∾ School change
- ∾ Divorce
- ∾ Change of religion
- ∾ Retirement
- ∾ Recovery from a long illness
- ∾ Disability
- ∾ Teething
- ∾ Puberty
- ∾ Menopause
- ∾ Midlife crisis
- ∾ Birth
- ∾ Death

People who need Walnut say about themselves:

- ∾ I'm planning to move, but I'm not completely happy about my new apartment.
- ∾ I want to quit my job and start something new. Yet I can't make up my mind completely, although inside of me I already have given notice.
- ∾ I'm in a phase of radical change in my life, but I haven't completely accepted the new.
- ∾ I still hang on to the old, although I want a new beginning.
- ∾ I feel insecure about everything new.

Mimulus and Larch people also suffer difficulties in a new situation. The following comparison will clarify the differences.

MINIMULUS	LARCH	WALNUT
Fear of new situations	Fear of making a fool of oneself; fear of failure	Cannot get along in new situations
Cause: fear	Cause: lack of self-esteem	Cause: inconstancy

Why is it that stable personalities and strong characters, who usually do not become insecure easily, also suffer from this inconstancy? Keep in mind that others are also affected by these changes and will therefore react to these actions. If, for example, a husband wants to change his job, his wife is affected by this plan as well, because she also risks suffering financial loss, lower social status, the loss of contact with other colleagues' wives, and so forth.

The Walnut individual not only wrestles with his own decision but also has to convince his family and friends. This implies the danger of becoming insecure through the well-meaning advice of others. Dominating social or moral conventions often make it difficult to translate formed decisions into action. Götz Blome therefore describes the Walnut state as the "conflict between our internal necessity and external pressure."[4]

Here Walnut can help one be true to one's self and to live and act according to one's beliefs. It protects one from disturbing external influences, provides a tough skin, and helps to withstand any influence and if necessary to swim against the current.

Like Centaury, Walnut also protects against subtle influences, for instance, in preventing sensitive healers from taking on their patients' symptoms. The action of Centaury, in contrast, is based more on the (often unnoticed) loss of energy to the environment. Centaury people often feel drained in the presence of low-energy people (for example, sick people) and suffer from unexplainable episodes of weakness.

Walnut also helps in periods of inner change, such as puberty and menopause, and for impulses that come from one's own inner self. It eases the emotional process of change that is necessary for the initiation of a new phase in life.

During puberty a girl changes into a woman. This transition often creates fear and can lead to physical symptoms that symbolize the inner conflict. Typical during this stage of life, acne represents the subconscious fear of the evolving sexuality. The face that is disfigured by pimples should appear unattractive to the opposite sex and should prevent an encounter with the fear-inducing new. Acne consequently protects one from confrontation with sexuality. The inner feeling of being torn between fascination and fear of something new, symbolized by the Scleranthus flower, often leads to the Crab Apple state, which is the decompensation of the Scleranthus phase. Sexuality is subsequently seen as something dirty. Sexual fantasies, unavoidable in this life phase, are seen as symptoms of inner impurity. This feeling is manifested in the form of skin disorders. Crab Apple in conjunction with Walnut is the main remedy for problems during puberty.

Disorders during menopause indicate that the change into a new phase in life has not been coped with emotionally. The loss of fertility is often associated with the loss of the feminine. This causes fear of losing one's attractiveness and of no longer being desirable to a man. The lower hormone production causes concern and the perception of not being sexually adequate. The body now tries to symbolize through heat flashes that the woman is still "hot." As the language of the body is not often understood, hormone treatments are prescribed; the heat flashes stop and the problem seems to be solved. This is an illusion, however, because the actual problem, the confrontation with one's own sexuality has still not happened on the emotional level. Rock Water is indicated in addition, if one tries to avoid the issue with a moral excuse of "We are past that age." To make a virtue out of necessity does not solve the problem but only leads to emotional rigidity.

For the strengthening the self-esteem in this difficult life stage, Larch is often needed.

Gorse *(Ulek europaeus)*

Gorse is the flower for those who after many failures have lost their faith when in seemingly impossible situations. In long chronic diseases, when no hope for recovery is left and the patient has lost all faith, Gorse is used. These people suffer from deep despair; everything seems to be gray and empty. They have already tried many things and by now have suffered so many drawbacks that they do not want to go on. Every further effort makes no sense to them, because they think that nothing can help them anymore. They no longer complain about their suffering, because even this seems to be useless. They are sometimes persuaded by their family members to try again, but they do so only as a favor. Deep inside they are already convinced of the uselessness of the endeavor.

Gorse people usually have a pale face with deep dark rings around their eyes. They say about themselves:

> ∾ Inside of me is a helpless, sad feeling; a feeling that no one can help me.
> ∾ I feel lost.

～ I feel completely desperate in this hopeless situation.

～ I feel inside like I'm stuck in the mire.

～ I'm incurably sick and have no more hope of recovery.

～ When I first heard the news, I was so desperate that I was afraid I would burst.

～ I'm a hopeless case.

～ No one has had as many infections as I have.

As a therapist it is hard to work with Gorse people. What can be done for individuals who themselves do not believe in their recovery or at least in the alleviation of their complaints, and who often do not even come out of their own free will? Their inner resentment represents the biggest obstacle on the road to health. One often gets the feeling that the treatment serves only as an alibi, and the expected failure is used to show the family proof of incurabilty. In this way the failure of the therapy is already preprogramed.

If there is, contrary to all expectations, a small success, the therapy will be terminated anyway, with the reason that the efforts are not worth the result. The patient has already gotten used to the idea of suffering for the rest of her life. In these cases Gorse can help to remove the internal blockage and to allow any sort of healing to take place, because the inner holding on to a disease is the actual cause of its incurability. Gorse acts as an emotional "retuning remedy"[5] and should be tried in chronic degenerative diseases in which recovery has come to a halt and the treatment has become stagnant.

Gorse has a certain resemblance to Gentian, Sweet Chestnut and Wild Rose. A comparison of the flowers' symptoms, in the succession of the intensity of despair, shows the differences clearly.

GENTIAN	GORSE	SWEET CHESTNUT	WILD ROSE
Easily discouraged, loses all hope very quickly.	Has lost courage, is without any hope, desperate.	Feels external despair, does not see a way out.	Feels resignation has capitulated to fate.
Does not believe in external help.	Gives up and waits for external help.	Feeling helpless, no longer knows what to do.	Has given up expecting anything from life.

A Sweet Chestnut state develops on the basis of a previously existing Agrimony state, in which all negativity is in principle ignored. By any means of distraction and escape into superficiality, a confrontation with problems and conflicts was avoided. The following compensatory Vervain state represents the attempt to escape inner sorrow of an extremely extraverted lifestyle. Finally, hit by a severe blow of fate, Sweet Chestnut people react with outer despair, as they already have endured extreme emotional pressure and are not able to tolerate it any longer.

A Wild Rose state is the result of previously existing Gentian and Willow states. Originating from a pessimistic attitude, in which those afflicted expect everything to be negative, they start to feel badly treated or even cheated by their own fate, which eventually leads to the circumstances they have quietly feared all along. Until now they have seen and expected only the negative side of things, so resignation remains the only thing left for them when these bad incidents finally occur.

A Gorse state, on the other hand, appears when there are repeated failures and hope for success ceases to exist.

Whether Agrimony people develop a Gorse or a Sweet Chestnut state in these situations depends on the emotional pressure they already had to bear during the Agrimony state, before the triggering circumstances. If they are already in a phase of compensation they might be inclined to the Sweet Chestnut state, in contrast to other Agrimony people, who will not reveal the big problems they hide.

Aspen *(Populus tremula)*

People who need Aspen suffer from vague indefinable fears. Some of them suffer from dark premonitions and imagine that a terrible disaster or catastrophe is about to happen. They get so involved in their irrational fear that they are virtually haunted by their own paranoia. In this way they turn their life into a living hell. Many of the things they are afraid of arise from their own fantasy; the infantile fear of ghosts is a typical example. The unreasonable fear of snakes and spiders also belongs to this category.

Aspen people say about themselves:

> ∾ I'm afraid of everything I can't touch directly with my hands.
> ∾ I suffer from irrational fears. In the past I was afraid of demons and dark forces.
> ∾ At night in my bed I often feel constriction in my chest and am terribly afraid, of what I don't know. I constantly feel afraid, especially of a recurrent panic attack at night.
> ∾ I'm often afraid of my own fear.
> ∾ When I'm alone I feel a terrible fear that is completely unreasonable.

- I often feel so frightened that I don't dare go outside.
- I'm frightened in the dark. Especially in the woods the darkness feels eerie to me.
- I always panic when I'm out on the street at night. Then I start running and it becomes creepier and creepier.
- Many times I wake up at night terribly frightened by nightmares.
- I'm afraid of ghosts.
- Sometimes I have the eerie feeling that someone is standing behind me.
- In the city I suddenly experience dizziness in connection with an unreasonable fear.
- I'm afraid of violent acts from men.
- I'm afraid of being raped.
- I bought myself a tear gas pistol because I'm afraid of being robbed.
- In the hospital I have a panicky fear that someone could poison me. The doctors think I suffer from an acute psychosis.
- I'm afraid I'll completely break down someday, although I'm absolutely healthy right now.
- I sometimes get the feeling something terrible has happened. Later, my apprehension turns out to be absolutely unsubstantiated; I had only imagined everything.
- When something bad happens to someone, I immediately fear that this could also happen to me. I can convince myself of many things.
- I'm afraid of the future.
- I'm often struck with terror that soon something bad will happen but I do not know what it might be.
- In some places I become extremely restless and fearful. Perhaps this has something to do with ground radiation or other negative vibrations. In some rooms there are spots where I can't stay.

Aspen has certain similarities with Rock Rose. Because a concrete reason for the fear exists in the latter, however, can be easily distinguished. The comparison of the flowers on the following page should show the differences more clearly.

The Aspen flower embodies the fear of all that is not comprehensible, especially things associated with religion and death. Aspen people are preoccupied with those topics and enhance their fear in this way.

ASPEN	ROCK ROSE
Irrational fear.	Fear as a result of a real experience.
Fear that something bad could happen.	Fear because something terrible has happened (accident, death of a family member, terrible disease, and so on).
Become scared by their own behavior and might even panic.	Are terribly frightened by an external event, start to panic, and out of fear are completely out of their minds.
Fear of the dark.	Start to panic because something in the dark frightens them.
Nightmares; are afraid of the things they have dreamt. The fear felt in the dream continues during the awake state. The fear of having another nightmare keeps them from falling asleep again.	Nightmares; awaken in a panic because they have experienced something horrible in their dreams. An accident or catastrophe is sometimes relived in the dream. The fear subsides shortly after being awakened by it.
Fear of physical violence, robbery, rape, abuse.	Fear during physical violence, robbery, rape, abuse.
Live in constant fear of imaginary things which can easily turn into panic through external events.	Chronic form: shock due to real experiences; shock and panic easily for no reason.

The image of Aspen is a mixture of fascination for occult phenomena and a simultaneous fear of them. They are fascinated by the eerie feeling, the goose bumps, and the chills going down their spines, all of which are proof for them that supernatural things exist. It is hard for them to let go of the fear, because they subconsciously fear losing the strangely attractive experience of occult phenomena.

Many of those afflicted feed their own fear because they gain some kind of pleasure out of the unknown. I know of one young man who visits graveyards in the middle of the night for this reason. Others lay cards, use the pendulum, or practice astrology out of the motivation to foresee accidents, disasters, or even catastrophes. They live with the constant fear of the fulfillment of their "prophecies." A colleague of mine, for example, does not drive his car if his horoscope indicates an accident danger; if a potential for an infection exists, he will not give injections on that day. Another example: a woman asked me in despair what she could do for her son; she had read in his horoscope that a terrible disaster would happen to him.

Aspen fears have an absolutely different character from those of Mimulus. In some cases it is not easy to determine whether the fear is vague or concrete; therefore the following comparison should help.

ASPEN	MINIMULUS
Vague fear, fear of the unknown.	Fear of unfamiliar things that can actually be named, such as new foods and strange surroundings on vacation.
Fear of the future, which looms threateningly; feeling of foreboding.	Fear of the future for specific reasons, such as financial problems, unemployment, debts.
Fear of death and what comes after.	Fear of dying, of the pain connected with it.
Irrational fear of robbery, physical violence.	Fear of burglars, that something will get stolen.
Infants who cry without a reason.	Infants who cry for a concrete reason, such as loud noises, bright light, and strange voices.

Such people easily become victims of their own delusions. The worst thing about it is that sometimes a disaster actually does happen to them. After all, there are "self-fulfilling prophecies"; the intense expectation of an event can make it happen. It does not even require negative thoughts, which according to the law of attraction would initiate the feared disaster in an invisible way. The individuals themselves can be the trigger through their own behavior.

For instance, in expectation of an accident a person might drive extra carefully and slowly. But this makes him a traffic hazard; he provokes other drivers to risky passing maneuvers, or causes a rear-end collision as he creeps in slow motion through an intersection. Once an accident happens, the prophecy has come true, and he views it as proof of his "seventh sense." Now every subsequent prophecy will be viewed as real. Because the motivation is fear, however, only the worst will be foreseen.

Such prophecies can have a catastrophic effect on relationships. If these people already predetermine the failure of a marriage they will desperately look for reasons. As a result of these "inspirations" they will make many unfounded accusations of their partners. Their behavior finally will provide the reason for the failure.

The Aspen type is extremely sensitive; some are even talented mediums. Herein exists a great danger, because a mediumistic gift in conjunction with fear can attract exactly those dark forces that they are afraid of. They will indeed experience fearful things: phenomena like obsession, frightening visions, sighting of demons, hallucinations, and so forth.

The Aspen state can be understood as the result of a subtle influence that the individual can feel but cannot classify. This perception subsequently creates a vague, indefinable fear. Just as touching a hot stove produces a burning pain that is recognized by the mind as heat, the perception of astral influences produces a feeling that we experience as fear because of the lack of detailed knowledge. Sensitive people explain that they felt frightened when they first perceived the so-called astral sphere, which they do not fear anymore because they now know these things and understand how to deal with them. This short sensation of fear serves for them as a distinctive signal of the connection with another dimension, similar to the burning pain that signals contact with a hot stove.

For this reason Aspen people are not served well by trying to talk them out of their fear, or by portraying their perceptions as hallucinations. Although they do imagine many things in their fear, their imagination is nevertheless based on "real" influences of an invisible, supernatural level of existence, of which they might not even be fully conscious. Because they cannot put these sensations into place but, as already mentioned above, perceive them as fear, they try to explain these unexplainable and eerie matters through their imagination. This (because of the extremity of the situation) triggers impulses and old fears that were stored in the subconscious. These become a blend of obsession and astral reality.

In this case it is important to explain the situation to the affected individuals—to the extent to which they are capable of and aware of the real background of their fear—and to help them to manage their sensitivity. The feeling of being misunderstood or being seen as crazy produces even more fear, especially if they think they have to handle those phenomena by themselves.

On the contrary, they have to learn to consciously free themselves from these "occult" phenomena, that is, to "look the other way." The practitioner must make clear to them that these astral influences will only do them harm if they open themselves up to them, will happens through fear. If they free themselves from these influences, all the appearances will fade away.

We are never completely alone. A whole cosmos of invisible vibrations constantly surrounds us. This is no reason to be afraid, however. Nature has limited our perception to the physical level so that we would not have to deal with other spheres all the time. Aspen people have to learn that there is no reason to panic if they perceive something from another sphere. They should try to distract themselves from these matters and to "look away," because their fear enhances their sensibility and provides the link to these perceptions.

An Aspen state in the extreme form as mentioned above is very rare but extremely dramatic. In the more frequent, milder version, the individuals complain about vague indefinable fears or fear of the dark. The mechanism in the origin of the fear, however, remains the same. The application of the Aspen flower will be sufficient to eliminate the fear. In more extreme Aspen states the counseling mentioned above is urgently needed, because otherwise the patient will sooner or later develop an acute psychosis.

6
RESCUE REMEDY

Rescue Remedy consists of a premixed Flower combination that can be applied as a first aid measure in emergencies of all kinds. The solution consists of the following flowers:

Star of Bethlehem for shock
Rock Rose for acute fear and panic
Impatiens for inner tension and stress
Cherry Plum for fear of breaking down in despair
Clematis for the feeling of being "not completely here"

The indication spectrum of this combination ranges from such emotional emergencies as acute fright or bad news to physical injuries, burns, and accidents. In cases of circulatory collapse and allergies it is the second remedy of choice (after medical emergency measures) to eliminate the fear that almost always occurs in these situations.

Rescue Remedy is always called for when a situation appears threatening to the individual or indeed might be life threatening. The state of shock paralyzes the energetic system; the conscious mind has the tendency to withdraw itself from the body or in extreme cases even to leave it. Psychics report that in these cases the so-called astral body partially or even completely separates from the physical body.

A friend experienced this event while fully conscious during a traffic accident. After the collision he looked down on the accident site and saw his badly injured body lying motionless among the wreckage of his motorcycle. In such cases the body is left completely on its own and is therefore unable to activate self-healing energy. The Rescue Remedy very quickly removes the energetic block and enables the body's regulatory system to initiate the necessary measures for emergencies. It is understandable, therefore, why this remedy has already saved many lives. In bad accidents and in life-threatening situations it serves as a practical first aid action until the physician has arrived.

An example will illustrate the rapid onset of the drop's action: A four-year-old boy who had knocked out his front teeth was bleeding profusely and screaming with pain. He immediately received a few drops of Rescue Remedy directly from the stock bottle on his tongue. Afterward he was given several Rescue Remedy drops and a homeopathic wound-healing remedy in a glass of water by drinking one sip every half minute. Ten minutes after the injury he fell asleep in his mother's arms. When he awoke several hours later the pain was completely gone.

Dr. Edward Bach used Rescue Remedy for the first time in 1930. It was then still in its original formula of Rock Rose, Clematis, and Impatiens; the two other flower ingredients he had not yet discovered. During a heavy storm off the coast of Cromer, the village in which Dr. Bach lived at that time, a small boat loaded with shingles shipwrecked. The crew, two men, clung to the mast of their sinking craft for many hours before a Coast Guard boat was able to rescue them. The younger of the two men had become unconscious, his face blue and his clothes stiff from the ocean salt. Dr. Bach ran into the water to meet the Coast Guard boat and moistened the sailor's lips with Rescue Remedy as he was carried out. He continued with the treatment all the way from the beach to the nearby hotel. Even before they had reached the hotel the unconscious man had regained consciousness, and even as they brought him in on a stretcher he asked for a cigarette.[1]

7

Discovering
the Appropriate Flower

The Interview
∞

The most important diagnostic instrument for finding the appropriate Bach Flower Remedy is the patient interview. All of the other diagnostic means represent only an addition to fill in the gaps of the interview and to complete the treatment plan. As in the title of Edward Bach's first German volume, Bach Flowers are, "Flowers that heal through the soul." Becoming aware of the emotional causes of momentary complaints through the patient interview is therefore of utter importance.

It also becomes clear that for the same reason a self-treatment cannot be very effective, except in acute existential disturbances, in which the negative emotional state is quite obvious. We always need a counterpart who is a sounding board for our problems. No one can be objective toward herself. Only the other person can make us aware of our inner faulty behavior, because she has the necessary distance from our problems.

Another important reason for the interview is the patients' need to be aware of the desired effect of the flowers on the psyche. This will prevent them from panicking if a potential reaction or a preliminary worsening of their symptoms occurs. The effect of the selected flowers should therefore be explained to them at the end of the session. In any case it is beneficial if they acquire some literature about Bach Flower Therapy so they can read about the different flower images at home.

The following questionnaire contains additional information about the respective flowers and enables the beginner to conduct a detailed interview without background knowledge. A copy of the questionnaire without this additional information can be found in the appendix of this book.

QUESTIONNAIRE

∾

1. Are there situations in which you are afraid?

Aspen:	vague, indefinable fear
Mimulus:	concrete fear
Rock Rose:	acute panic
Cherry Plum:	fear of going crazy, freaking out
Red Chestnut:	worrying about other people
Larch:	expectation anxiety, fear of failure or of making a fool of oneself
Centaury:	fear of not being acknowledged
Crab Apple:	fear of infections

2. Are there situations in which you feel insecure?

Cerato:	I often ask other people for advice in decision making
Scleranthus:	every problem has two possibilities
Wild Oat:	too many options, therefore confused; I don't know what I want
Gentian:	I doubt everything; easily discouraged
Gorse:	without hope; I don't believe in help anymore
Hornbeam:	mentally exhausted; I question my own strength

3. Do you sometimes lack concentration? Are you easily distracted from your work?

Clematis:	daydreamer; I live in a fantasy world
Honeysuckle:	I live in the past
White Chestnut:	I can't relax; annoying thoughts
Chestnut Bud:	I'm always two steps ahead in my mind
Wild Rose:	no interest, indifferent, lackadaisical
Mustard:	melancholic, unexplainable sadness
Olive:	exhausted, absolutely devastated

4. Do you sometimes feel lonely?

Heather:	I very quickly feel lonely; always need someone around
Water Violet:	withdraw to the inside; difficulties making contact

Impatiens: I would rather work alone; no one can keep up with my work speed

5. In what situations are you influenced by others?

Centaury: can't say no; lack of own will

Walnut: in a phase of new beginning, therefore fickle

Holly: I get mad quickly; easily irritated

Agrimony: entertainer; I tend to take alcohol or drugs

6. Are there situations in which you feel discouraged or desperate?

Star of Bethlehem: after an emotional shock, accident, death in the family

Sweet Chestnut: absolutely desperate; I believe I will fall apart from suffering

Willow: I feel unfairly treated, embittered

Crab Apple: I perceive myself as unclean, condemn myself for my alleged sins

Larch: I perceive myself as less efficient and capable; I lack self-esteem

Elm: I feel temporarily not strong enough to do a specific task; overwhelmed; for example, before examinations

Oak: I'm exhausted, but continue to work on out of a sense of duty; drained

7. Do you worry about the well-being of other people?

Chicory: overprotective character

Vine: I know everything better and force my will on others

Beech: I think I have to point out other people's mistakes, criticize, and reproach

Vervain: I believe I can convince everyone of my ideas; missionary zeal

Rock Water: strict moral ideas; I want to be an example for others

8. To what do you react sensitively?

Mimulus: loud noises, bright light, cold, other people's aggression

Agrimony: environmental disturbances, for example, noisy children, music, soft noises

Larch: to criticism and reproach, because of lack of self-esteem

Pine:	to accusations, which make me feel guilty
Vervain:	injustice
Impatiens:	people who work slower; slow-driving cars that I can't pass
Centaury:	resentment, the feeling of not being accepted, suffering people, because of a strong empathy
Gentian:	failure, because I am easily discouraged
Chicory:	ingratitude, unpleasant and rude behavior of others

9. What do you think about, when you have time to think?

Star of Bethlehem:	unpleasant things in the past
Honeysuckle:	pleasant things in the past
Clematis:	fantasies, daydreams, plans for the future
White Chestnut:	I can't stop thinking
Willow:	injustice done to me
Chestnut Bud:	what I will do next
Red Chestnut:	about others, whether they are doing well

10. What makes you angry?

Holly:	everything; I get angry very easily
Centaury:	myself because I can't say no
Vervain:	myself when I don't fulfill my own expectations
Rock Water:	myself after I go against my conscience or after I ignore my own rules
Beech:	the stupidity of other people.
Impatiens:	having to wait

11. What is dissatisfying to you?

Chicory:	my son or daughter-in-law; ingratitude
Wild Oat:	I can't find my goal in life; I don't know what to do; I have no perspective.
Vervain:	myself; too high expectations of myself
Pine:	the mistakes I've made; guilt feelings
Rock Water:	that I don't live up to my morals
Impatiens:	everything goes too slowly
Hornbeam:	that I'm too exhausted to be productive
Water Violet:	everything is too banal; I look for special things, because I think of myself as being superior.

12. What makes you feel exhausted?

Olive:	total physical and psychological exhaustion after illness or phases of colossal overwork

Hornbeam:	mental exhaustion after too much intellectual work, studying or reading at night
Elm:	sudden exhaustion, blackout
Oak:	I'm overworked, but I continue to work out of a sense of duty
Centaury:	I'm drained by the presence of other people, overworked by too much helpfulness

13. What keeps you from being completely happy?

Holly:	anger
Willow:	bitterness
Wild Oat:	no perceivable goals
Wild Rose:	everything appears meaningless; I've given up
Gorse:	desperate; no one can help me
Sweet Chestnut:	deep despair; I'm without hope
Pine:	guilt feelings
Crab Apple:	feel dirty on the inside, sinful, soiled
Rock Water:	repressed desires
Vervain:	I can be happy only if I meet my own expectations
Star of Bethlehem:	emotional trauma
Scleranthus:	a sudden drop from seventh heaven to deadly depression
Gentian:	pessimism, exogenous reactive depression
Mustard:	unexplainable, endogenous depression
Water Violet:	I've withdrawn from life; I'm above the simple pleasures of life
Agrimony:	I appear to be lighthearted to the outside
Hornbeam:	I'm too exhausted to feel joy about something
Olive:	I'm absolutely exhausted, thinking only of sleep

14. Do you sometimes feel sad and blue?

Mustard:	unexplainable endogenous depression
Gentian:	known reason for sadness, exogenous reactive depression
Wild Oat:	I don't see a meaning or a goal in life
Gorse:	sad, without hope
Sweet Chestnut:	absolute despair

15. Are you careless about minor details or are you a perfectionist?

Careless, sloppy:

Wild Rose:	because of resignation

Wild Oat: because nothing has meaning

Clematis: because of lack of attention; my thoughts are somewhere else

Chestnut Bud: I postpone unpleasant tasks, many things appear unimportant to me

Water Violet: I feel I am above the existing order; "those who need order are too lazy to search—the genius has a general overview"; in certain areas, on the other hand, I'm a perfectionist

Heather: in children: to get attention, even if this means disciplining or spanking for them

Hornbeam: because of exhaustion, although this is usually not my nature

Mustard: because of a feeling of an inner emptiness, only during melancholic phases

Perfectionist:

Crab Apple: I have to do everything perfectly, otherwise I feel unclean; compulsive perfection

Vervain: with enthusiasm, combined with extremely high self-expectations; I want to prove myself

Rock Water: I'm an idealist; I try to prove my point to other people by being a role model

Water Violet: I want to be better than others to justify my feelings of superiority; I'm sloppy, however, in daily affairs

Heather: to be the center of attention; I need an audience

Centaury: to be liked by others

16. Do you mind if you have to wait?

Impatiens: I'm impatient

Cherry Plum: I'm afraid of going crazy (especially in people who take drugs)

Holly: I'm angry

Beech: I complain to other people about the person who made me wait

Gentian: I'm afraid that it is too late for my turn

17. Do you frequently make the same mistakes?

Chestnut: I don't learn from my mistakes

Clematis: I don't pay attention; I dream a lot

Centaury: I'm always fooled by the same trick, I can't say no

18. Do you sometimes have the feeling that you are superior to other people?

> Water Violet: I think of myself as better than others
> Rock Water: in a moral sense; I perceive other people as heathens, sinners

19. Do you tend to have feelings of guilt?

> Pine: I feel guilty
> Crab Apple: I perceive myself as unclean, sinful, and soiled

20. Do you feel jealousy and envy?

> Holly: jealousy, envy

21. Do you feel you have been unfairly treated by somebody else? Is there someone whom you cannot forgive? Do you know the feeling of bitterness?"

> Willow: embittered; I feel like a victim

22. Do you sometimes feel unclean in some way? Are you bothered by dirt? Do you feel disgusted by other people's toilets? Do you feel disgusted by spiders and snakes?"

> Crab Apple: fear of dirt, infection, sweat; disgust with every thing having to do with the body

23. Is it sometimes hard for you to make a decision? How do you behave when you have to make a decision?

> Cerato: I need confirmation through others
> Scleranthus: I can't decide between two options; I feel torn
> Wild Oat: I can't decide among several options
> Walnut: I feel insecure in a new phase in my life, therefore, I can't make decisions
> Hornbeam: I often can't decide to get out of bed

24. Are you more of an optimist or a pessimist?

> Gentian: pessimist
> Agrimony: I pretend to be an optimist, but I'm tortured by sorrows

25. Do you sometimes wish you had more self-esteem? Can you speak in public to an audience?

> Larch: lack of self-esteem
> Cerato: lack of trust in my own ability to judge; I ask other people for advice
> Centaury: lack of will; I can't say no

26. How do you assert yourself in your environment? What do you do when other people have a completely different opinion from yours? What would you do if you had to do something that you resent with all your heart?

Vervain:	try to convince others
Vine:	try violence, threaten with consequences
Chicory:	use the diplomatic approach; tell the others what has already been done for them and that they should be grateful
Impatiens:	try to resolve the matter as soon as possible, and often overreact because of my impatience
Rock Water:	stick to my principles; under extreme circumstances I'd even risk my job

27. How do you react to unpleasant things?

Anger:

Holly:	I react impulsively; I yell at others; I have a difficult time calming down again; I'm resentful
Centaury:	I'm quick to give in to "maintain the peace"
Water Violet:	I withdraw; I look at hassles as beneath my dignity
Beech:	I reproach others, look for mistakes, try to hurt other people with my clever remarks
Larch:	I can't easily defend myself; low self-esteem

Sorrow:

Heather:	I wail and lament
Star of Bethlehem:	I'm shocked
Agrimony:	I deal with my problem alone; I don't speak to anyone about my problems; I try to move on
Gentian:	I'm easily discouraged; I give up
Gorse:	I feel desperate

28. Do you like to be comforted when you are sad?

Agrimony:	I deal with everything myself
Heather:	I have a deep desire for solace

29. Do you solve your problems on your own or with the help of others?

Alone:

Agrimony:	I don't admit my problems; cheerful facade
Water Violet:	I'm too proud to accept help

With others:

Cerato: I ask other people for advice

Heather: I need a shoulder to cry on

30. Are there things you consciously avoid because they go against your general principles?

Rock Water: I'm focused on my principles; I suppress my own desires

31. Are you a good listener, or do you sometimes take over a conversation?

Vervain: I want to convince other people

Heather: I direct attention to myself; I need an audience; I can't listen very well

Impatiens: in my impatience I interrupt other people

32. What do you worry about?

Heather: about myself; hypochondriac

Red Chestnut: about other people, that something might happen to them

Chicory: I watch over the needs of others; overprotective

Gentian: about the future; I like to worry

33. Have you ever been without hope, resigned? Did you ever in your life give up?

Gentian: easily discouraged, doubtful

Gorse: desperate; I believe no one can help me

Sweet Chestnut: deepest despair; I see absolutely no way out; I'm completely at the end of my rope

Wild Rose: resignation, inner capitulation

34. Have you ever had experiences that shocked you?

Star of Bethlehem: emotional shock, emotional trauma

Rock Rose: fright, panic, mortal fear

35. Do you have thoughts that you can't let go of and that constantly occupy you? Do you talk to yourself sometimes?

White Chestnut: I can switch off my thoughts

Chestnut Bud: I'm always two steps ahead in my thoughts

Clematis: fantasies, daydreams

Pine: tormenting thoughts; I make excuses for myself

36. Are there situations that weigh heavily on you?
In what kinds of situations do you feel tense?

Impatiens: impatient, nothing goes fast enough

Vervain: I want to convince other people, therefore I have a hard time letting go; I'm unable to relax

Agrimony: inner nervousness when going to sleep, worried thoughts

Oak: I often work beyond my limits until I reach my second wind; therefore I'm totally tense

Rock Water: I frantically hold on to my moral values

Cherry Plum: constant inner tension, so as not to lose control

Beech: I always have to criticize something; my constant negativity makes me emotionally hard

37. Are there situations in which you react intolerantly?

Beech: in all situations; I moan and lecture

Impatiens: if someone is slower than me

Rock Water: against a different ideology, I don't accept anything else, I'm intolerant of my own desires.

Vervain: against another opinion; I try to convince others

Heather: I'm absolutely egocentric; I don't let other people talk; I want to be the center of attention

Holly: I don't put up with anything; I'm aggressive

38. What annoys you the most? What would you most like to change about yourself?

PARTNER DIAGNOSIS

In the interview some patients constantly complain about other people. Whether it is the mean mother-in-law, the tyrannical boss, the bad neighbors, the naughty children, or even his own wife—it is always someone else who is to blame for his own bad luck. It is most often his own behavior, however, that offers the other person the opportunity to influence him in one way or the other.

Make use of those complaints for your diagnosis. Let the patient describe in detail the person who occupies his thoughts. You can draw from it important conclusions about the patient's own character. It doesn't matter who that person really is. Every individual who in some way or another represents a partner to the patient, as in the private or professional area, is suitable because that person holds a mirror up to the patient's face and forces him to react. Therefore, it does not have to be the marital partner but can also be the business partners, who—through their behavior—can trigger a reaction or feelings that put them into the center of the patient's life.

Some examples should show how a virtual symbiosis with other persons is formed in this way, which in many cases can be painful for the weaker partner. If the patient describes his partner as tyrannical and domineering, one has to ask why he goes along and doesn't resist. Vine people need a Centaury partner to live out their drive for power.

Chicory people who constantly emphasize what they have already done for other people and how much they are owed by them often create guilt feelings. When a Chicory partner is mentioned in the interview—no matter if it is the spouse, mother, or employer—one should always think of Pine. Children of Chicory people almost always suffer from guilt.

For Heather people, who immediately have to pass on everything that has happened to them and moved them, who always need an audience and cannot let go of someone once they have grabbed them, only good-natured Centaury partners can be good listeners, because they have the willpower to resist the assertive behavior of Heather people.

Vervain people, who in their euphoria try to convince everyone around them of their ideas, need Cerato partners who can listen to them. Vice versa, Cerato people are usually happy when they find someone who is willing to give them pieces of information, since they look for advice because of their inner insecurity.

There are also flower types, who look not for a complementary partner but rather for someone with the exact same flaws. Götz Blome writes: "Agrimony is an equal-minded partner remedy, as this type of personality can be lived only if the partner acts in a similar fashion. The artificiality of Agrimony people can be accepted only by people of their own kind, because only someone who lives on the surface will like it if his counterpart stays on the periphery as well. It is a prearranged game, as if onstage."[1]

Beech is also a like-minded partner remedy. If this relationship is a harmonic partnership, both people will enjoy scoffing at other people. If, however, the partnership is disharmonious, they will criticize and yell at each other and complain about each other's intolerance. Those who complain about the intolerance of the other person are usually also intolerant, otherwise they would not be bothered by it at all.

Diagnosis through the Language of the Organs

∾

Physical symptoms, according to Edward Bach, are the manifestation of negative thoughts. Therefore, it makes sense to use the physical complaints to find the needed flowers. We just have to learn to understand the "language" of the body and to interpret the symptoms correctly. The following possibilities are available.

1. Idioms or popular sayings can give us clues about the connection between an emotional state and the corresponding organ. Examples:

Heart:	This broke my heart. His heart is as cold as ice.
Stomach:	This is hard to digest.
Thyroid:	This is hard to swallow.
Head:	This gives me a headache.
Eyes:	You can't just look the other way. What I don't see can't hurt me.
Spine:	He has no backbone.
Skin:	This got under my skin.
Blood vessels:	This made my blood freeze.

2. Freudian slips can also be deduced from the organ functions. Examples:

The legs serve as a mode of transportation. Complaints in this area (for example, in the knee or hip joints) indicate that one wants to run away from something.

The skin is the point of contact between us and our environment. Skin disorders often symbolize problems in making contact. The texture of the skin gives clues about the particular kind of problem. Psoriasis indicates that the patient created a "strong shield" for herself; she likes to separate herself from her environment.

Emptying the bladder is a passive act that works through the relaxation of the bladder's sphincter muscles. Disturbances in this body function symbolize that a patient cannot let go. A bladder infection or painful urination shows that letting go is felt as something painful.

Waste products are eliminated through the colon. Constipation symbolizes that a patient does not want to give up something but is frantically trying to hold on to it. Diarrhea indicates fear of failure (test anxiety) or losing the recognition of other people.

3. Through the type of body reaction it is also possible to draw conclusions about emotional flaws. Examples:

In the case of an infection the body's own immune system "fights" invading "enemies" such as bacteria, viruses, or fungi. Every infection represents a militant confrontation on the level of the body's own immune system. Thorwald Dethlefsen writes: "Each infection is a materialized conflict. Confrontation that was avoided in the psyche (with all its pain and dangers) forces itself onto the physical level for acknowledgment."[2]

In cases of allergies, the body's own immune system fights against harmless substances such as pollen or house dust. The body does not "tolerate" these substances and resists vehemently. The aggression shows itself in the form of infections, inflammations, itching, sneezing, and can even take on a life-threatening form in the case of anaphylaxis.

In the case of the rheumatic illnesses, the body is destroying itself. The fighting cells attack the body's own cells instead of invading pathogens. Depending on the disease, the bones, soft tissue, or blood vessels are affected. Medicine talks about "autoaggression." It stands symbolically for the aggression that has not been overtly lived, but instead is directed against oneself.

Each lingering feeling of hate produces a rising infection process in the body. The aggression has to be worked out on the physical level if one always swallows one's anger instead of letting it out or looking for a solution to the problem. Everything we do not want to live out in our psyche we shall meet again in our body as a symptom. We cannot run away from the lessons of life; our bodies prevent this from happening by making us painfully aware of them on a physical level and thereby forcing us to look for solutions to our problems.

The language of the organs can help us track down the emotional reasons for our ailments. It is not possible, however, to relate certain diseases to the flowers. Only the particular quality of the symptoms can give us clues about what might be going on in the patient's psyche. There is, for example, no flower for hypotension. Still, people with low blood pressure usually do not feel strong enough to withstand the burden of daily life, therefore Hornbeam automatically comes to mind. Wild Rose could also be considered in the case of a physically manifested resignation.

The above-mentioned symptoms of an infection remind us of Holly. The allergy as an expression of physical intolerance indicates Beech, whereas the autoaggression carries clear signs of Willow characteristics. These analogies should only be seen as hints, however, and need to be confirmed by the interview with the patient.

DIAGNOSIS THROUGH THE BACH FLOWER BODY MAPS

∾

This diagnosis is much easier than the one through organ language. No interpretation is necessary that would require detailed knowledge about psychosomatic or body language. The zones of the flowers are predetermined, similar to the foot reflex zones. It is therefore possible to "read" directly from the body what flower remedy is needed for the particular disturbances of these zones. The topography covers the whole body.

There are two categories taken into consideration for the zones:

1. Painful areas on the body are always disturbed. In this way the applicable flower remedy can be determined just through localizing the complaints.
2. There are also "silent" zones, which—although disturbed—do not create any complaints "at this site." They can be found through sensitive diagnostic methods.

There are correlations between the painful and the "silent" zones, according to the corresponding tracks. The suitable "silent" zones can be deduced through interpretation and are consequently also available for practitioners who cannot or do not want to make a sensitive diagnosis.

The skin zones are the focus of my second book, *New Bach Flower Body Maps,* where I describe them in conjunction with the diagnosis of the aura and the corresponding therapeutic opportunities.

ASTROLOGICAL DIAGNOSIS

∾

At the beginning of Bach Flower Therapy, astrological views were always kept in mind. Edward Bach himself appeared to be convinced of astrology's value, although he did not want to make a decisive statement until this method was proved. In 1933 he wrote in a letter that he decided not to include astrological information in *The Twelve Healers* because the correlations between astral signs and flower essences were not yet conclusively determined. As long as his results were still vague, he felt, they were not ready for publication.[3]

Peter Damian has rediscovered this theme and published it in a simple and accessible way. His book *The Twelve Healers of the Zodiac* describes a simple method for the flower diagnosis based on the horoscope, which can be practiced even by an astrological layperson. Damian based his findings on Bach's writings, which classify the first twelve remedies Bach discovered as the main remedies and the later ones as supplemental. Those main remedies, first introduced in the pamphlet *The Twelve Healers* in 1933, were obviously associated at the time to the twelve zodiac signs, as the above-cited letter indicates.

Afterward, Bach discovered seven more flower remedies and named them the "Seven Helpers." In 1935 he wrote in a letter to a colleague that each of the subsequently discovered remedies corresponded to one or another of the Twelve Healers or Seven Helpers. For example, if a Clematis case develops well but does not heal completely, then one of the later remedies will induce the healing."[4]

For this reason, Peter Damian uses only the flowers first discovered by Bach in his astrological method. The twenty-six other flowers are defined by him as supplemental flowers; only to be used when indicated.

In my system the "twelve healers" correspond to the Communication flowers and can also be calculated astrologically according to Damian's system. Because each of these flowers is associated with two more flowers, a total of thirty-two flowers—which I have named the inner flowers—can be incorporated into the astrological diagnosis. Of the remaining six flowers, the five outer flowers are remedies for the actions and effects of external influences and therefore cannot be incorporated into the astrological concept. The foundation flower, Larch, is used only according to the indication and therefore is independent from other flowers or astrological circumstances.

Damian includes seven criteria in his astrological diagnosis:

1. The position of *the Sun* during birth symbolizes the basic personality traits. It represents self-esteem, assertion, endurance, individual life force, and energy; it correlates to our masculine side.

2. *The Ascendant* symbolizes our individuality and therefore our external image in our environment. It shows us our temperament and the way we solve our problems and approach the tasks life has to offer us. The ascendant shows the degree of the ecliptic that ascends at the time of birth on the eastern horizon. Because all the zodiac signs ascend within twenty-four hours, it is possible to make much more individual statements about a person than with the Sun, which only changes its position in the zodiac only once a month.

3. *The Moon* represents our emotional world, our desires, and our passion. It represents our feminine, passive side and consequently the unconscious. Edward Bach writes in *The*

Twelve Healers that our personality reveals itself to us in the constellation of the moon at our birth, but that we must not put too much emphasis on the planets; if we stay with our personality and remain faithful to ourselves, we need not worry about planetary or external influences. The remedies can help us stand up for our personality.[5]

4. *Mercury* symbolizes our mental temperament, that is, our intellectual capabilities, our mind. It represents both rational comprehension and logical thinking as well as the thirst for knowledge, enthusiasm and goal setting, which are mental activities. Peter Damian suggests that Mercury offers clues about one's own thought patterns, an important factor, since the flowers affect the mental constitution.[6]

5. *Saturn* embodies the human desire for protection and security. For this reason we set up protective borders, which, however, limit us and make our lives more difficult. Consequently, Saturn becomes the symbol for restriction and limitation. It shows us our weak points and obstacles on our way through life. Fear is also connected with *Saturn,* because constriction and limitation of our freedom automatically generate fear.

6. *The First House* as the symbol for the "I" (starting with the ascendant) shows the basis of people, as much on the mental level (for example, character traits, willpower) as on the physical one (for example, postures and features of the physical body, constitution, and physical flaws).

7. *The Ruling Planet of the Ascendant* can be found with the help of the graph on the following page:

It proved valuable in my work to incorporate the medium coeli (or midheaven) and the ascending moon node whereas the ascendant portrays us as we are seen by others, the medium coeli symbolizes the real personality that we should develop during our lives. It also stands for vocation and life destination. The ascending moon node, on the other hand represents our tasks on the way there. An exact interpretation according to the teaching of astrological psychology offers even more precise clues than the more preliminary method Damian suggests for laypeople.

Many inexpensive computer programs are available for calculating horoscopes on a personal computer. If you do not want to bother with calculating your horoscope yourself, you can have yours done through one of the many astrological services. Once you have your horoscope in hand, the technique for astrological analysis according to Damian is simple. In the horoscope you look up the ascendant and its ruling planet, along with the signs in which lie the Sun, the Moon, Mercury, and Saturn. If there is a planet in the first house, that is not in the same astrological sign as the ascendant, add this sign as well.

ZODIAC SIGN	RULING PLANET
Aries	Mars
Taurus	Venus
Gemini	Mercury
Cancer	Moon
Leo	Sun
Virgo	Mercury
Libra	Venus
Scorpio	Pluto/Mars
Sagitarius	Jupiter
Capricorn	Saturn
Aquarius	Uranus/Saturn
Pisces	Neptune/Jupiter

Horoscope Example

The data table is used for interpretation only. A classification of the horoscope is not necessary. In this way the astrological newcomer does not need to learn the astrological signs and symbols.

The numbers in parentheses indicate the position in the respective house. In the calculation Koch houses are used because this is customary in astrological psychology.

Name: Fritz Muster
Date of Birth: April 25, 1951
Time of Birth: 5.30 P.M.
Place of Birth: Frankfurt, Germany
Longitude: 8°41'
Latitude: 50°07'
Houses: Koch

Ascendant:	13°40'	Libra
Sun:	4°40'	Taurus (7)
Moon:	27°2'	Sagittarius (3)
Mercury:	3°48'	Taurus (7)

Venus:	12°12'	Gemini (9)
Mars:	11°18'	Taurus (7)
Jupiter:	0°55'	Aries (6)
Saturn:	26°28'	Virgo (12)
Uranus:	6°11'	Cancer (9)
Neptune:	17°43'	Libra (1)
Pluto:	17°25'	Leo (11)
Moon Node:	16°43'	Pisces (6)

The seven-step analysis according to Peter Damian[7] yields the following:

1. Sun in Taurus
2. Ascendant in Libra
3. Moon in Sagittarius
4. Mercury in Taurus
5. Saturn in Virgo
6. Neptune is located in the first house. Because this is the same sign as the Ascendant, we do not have to take it into consideration.
7. Ruler of the Ascendant is Venus, in Gemini
   Result: Taurus, Libra, Sagittarius, Virgo, Gemini

The astrological diagnosis thus indicates the corresponding flower remedies for these five astrological signs.

The classification of the Bach Flowers to the individual zodiac signs according to Peter Damian is as follows:

Aries:	Impatiens
Taurus:	Gentian
Gemini:	Cerato
Cancer:	Clematis
Virgo:	Centaury
Libra:	Scleranthus
Scorpio:	Chicory
Sagittarius:	Agrimony
Capricorn:	Mimulus
Aquarius:	Water Violet
Pisces:	Rock Rose

The outcome in our example would be the following five communication flowers: Gentian, Scleranthus, Agrimony, Centaury, and Cerato.

According to Damian's directions, all five remedies should be given whether the client accepts them or not. Damian reasons that although no one is completely honest with himself, the horoscope will tell the truth in any case and should therefore be seen as more objective than the client's statement.

If any other flowers are needed (as a result of the interview), they should be given in a separate bottle and in alternation with the astrological solution, for example, one solution before dinner and one after. According to Damian, but contrary to the recommendation of the Dr. Bach Center, it does not matter if more than six or seven different flowers are given simultaneously. Often, according to this method, ten to twelve flowers may be necessary.

I myself have practiced for a long time according to this method and have come to the following results: When I add the astrological solution to the one found through the interview a significantly increased effectiveness could be noted. The patient often reported intense dreams to a degree that he or she had never before experienced. When I applied only the astrological remedy—without the flowers found necessary by the patients—either nothing happened or unpleasant reactions occurred (for example, an increase in the existing symptoms or a feeling of inner agitation). The actual complaints, however, did not get better. The exceptions were cases in which the astrologically diagnosed remedies had also been found through the interview.

First of all, those reactions brought me to the conclusion that the astrological solution serves as a kind of catalyst that can enhance the effect of the different flower combinations or eliminate existing blocks in therapy. If we give the "catalyst" on its own it only leads to reactions, with no improvement of the symptoms.

A completely different result is achieved through the work with the tracks. If we compare the flowers found astrologically with the ones given according to the symptoms, we notice the following:

1. Some of the flowers found in the horoscope are also ascertained by the interview.
2. Some flowers that apply to the symptoms of compensation or decompensation are also found through the astrological method.
3. For some astrologically determined flowers, no other ones of the same track are seen by the client to be applicable.
4. For many compensation and decompensation flowers ascertained in the interview, the corresponding communication flower cannot be found in the horoscope.

Regarding 1. This needs no comment, except that it does not happen often. If it were the rule, we could indeed substitute the long interview with the horoscope (with a computer, the astrological interpretation takes approximately five minutes altogether).

Regarding 2. This is the ideal case. The horoscope reveals the fundamental emotional cause for the momentary problems, which often are unknown to the individuals, as we have already seen in the description of the individual communication flowers. Furthermore, the suffering becomes evident only in the stages of compensation or decompensation, in which the subconscious inner conflict first manifests itself as a problem.

Regarding 3. If one accepts the astrological statements as facts, only one conclusion can be made in a case when the astrologically discovered flower does not have an effect: the (astrologically postulated) problem is not an acute one. Consequently, there is no reason to use that flower for an acute problem; if anything, it would be a hindrance.

Regarding 4. Obviously it is impossible to calculate life in advance. After all, we are able, thanks to our free will, to interfere actively with our destiny and to fend off the unavoidable as much as to look for new lessons. It is this free will that makes any dogmatic application of astrology fail. Nevertheless, astrology can be a valuable tool in the hands of therapists, as long as they "play by the rules."

Especially in children, with whom an interview is not possible and one has to rely on the observation of the parents, an astrological interpretation offers valuable clues. The question that arises sometimes is, Who actually has problems with whom—the parents with the child or the child with the parents?

For me, astrological psychology is a diagnostic tool similar to the iridology. It reveals the emotional qualities of people, their strong and weak points and the possible conflicts and arguments that might evolve from them. It shows—speaking in a metaphor—what kind of horses we have in the stall. We are free to decide which one we want to ride most. Therefore, we should always ask ourselves when doing astrological flower diagnosis: What lesson does the individual want to learn *right now?* What emotional concept from the horoscope does he or she live in *right now?*

Astrology shows us the background, but the interview with the patient still provides us with the main criteria for the selection of the flowers. Astrology, though, points us to the direction we have to go and thereby prevents us from overlooking an essential fact. I believe that in this function lies the main value of astrology.

One important clue was given by Edward Bach himself: he thought that the constellation of the moon was of utter importance. My own observation can only verify this. Most often the main problem shows itself in the position of the moon, the ascendant, or both. The position of the sun—contrary to one's assumption—is not of great importance.

In my experience it has been proven best to do the astrological interpretation prior to the interview and to transcribe the result into the flow sheet. In this way certain connections become more obvious during the interview, and I have the possibility to ask more in-depth questions at certain points. One should pay special attention to the flowers that belong to the positions of the moon and the ascendant.

The most important chance to learn can be recognized when the patient is in the phase of decompensation, which corresponds with the points 2 and 4 above. Flowers described under point 3 should be disregarded. In my opinion only flowers that are seen by the individual as the right ones should be used. If one still wants to use them, special consent from the patient should be obtained.

When patients refuse a particular flower, it may be because they are either unaware of the main problem or they do not want to learn that lesson. Because it is not allowed for us to interfere with anyone's free will, we should not give these flowers to them without their consent.

Once the actual problems have faded and no further flower remedy is necessary for them, it is possible to use the flowers described under point 3 on a trial basis, if desired by the patient. The practitioner, however, must be convinced that those flowers are suited. One should certainly be very careful in the approach; it could come to vehement reactions in the treatment of character flaws that have been unknown to the individuals so far.

With the flower Clematis, for example, it is possible to help people with Mercury in Cancer to live more in the here and now. Their pleasant dwelling in their daydreams has perhaps not caused any problems for them so far, and they may therefore perceive this state as absolutely normal. Mercury in Cancer, though, indicates a possibility to pursue their work with more concentration and to experience reality more clearly and consciously. Because drifting off in fantasies during unpleasant situations will cease through the application of Clematis, a painful awakening can occur, which under certain circumstances can even lead to short-term depressions. On the other hand, when Clematis is used for people who suffer from their fantasies (e.g., who develop headaches because they constantly have to force themselves to work), the above described reactions do not occur; instead the patients experience significant relief.

If we want to use the Bach Flowers to expand our consciousness, in principle we should first consider any communication flowers that correspond to compensation and decompensation flowers that have already been applied especially if the communication flower has not been used so far because it did not seem suitable. This path of treatment makes sense, because such flowers represent the (unconscious) causes of already treated complaints. The astrologically ascertained flowers in point 3 above are therefore good at the end of a treatment as well, if we choose to use them at all.

Astrology applied in the right way can help us to choose the right Bach Flower Remedies. We should always be aware of the fact, however, that life really symbolizes a school in which each needed flower is a lesson. The horoscope shows us the individual "lesson plan." Life can accept spontaneous lessons, though, if the circumstances seem to be favorable. The lesson already learned cannot be taken out of the curriculum. The more we work on ourselves, however, the further away we move from our horoscope.

OTHER DIAGNOSTIC METHODS

The *Bioelectronic Function Diagnostic* (BFD) measures the resistance of the skin between acupuncture points. In the wire between the point probe and the electronic device a small aluminium honeycomb is placed, in which small bore holes are located for the installation of vials or little medicine bottles. If a medication is placed inside this circuit, it is possible to determine from the change of skin resistance whether a certain remedy agrees with the patient or not. This technique is not as easy as one might think at first glance, however, and requires a great deal of experience to achieve reproducible results.

The *Touch for Health* is a muscle test in which the test person extends the arm upward with all his strength, while the therapist tries to push down the arm. Here the resistance is tested that is met by the external force. If the test person takes a medication in his hand, the resistance changes. Because the body subconsciously reacts to the vibrations of the medication, the test preson will withstand the counterforce better or worse, depending on whether the remedy agrees or disagrees with him.

In trials of both methods I was able to observe that the test indicates only the superficial flower remedies. The deeper psychological background found through the interpretation of the tracks could not be determined by these mechanical methods. Whatever a patient is unaware of on the conscious level he also does not "know" on the physical level. It is therefore impossible to recall this information through measuring techniques—of any kind—that are oriented toward the body.

Moreover, I do not find it very meaningful to apply substances that work in the emotional realm only because of some physical measurement. The same is true for the use of pendulums for Bach Flowers. A manipulation of the psyche without the individual's being aware of the consequences represents a massive interference with the free will.

Therefore, Bach Flower Therapy without a detailed interview is unthinkable. Patients need to become aware of what they would like to change before those changes can be initiated through the Bach Flower Remedies, and the interview makes that possible.

In acute cases, the other diagnostic methods, especially the *Touch for Health,* can be of some benefit to the beginner after the interview when it is difficult to decide between two flowers. A review of the particular flower portraits, however, might also offer more clarity, so that it may be a better use of time to study the different flower images rather than with mechanical methods.

Some practitioners set the remedies in front of the patients so that they are not able to read the labels. They then ask them to pick the bottles spontaneously. I do not use this method of *intuitive drawing* because in my opinion it moves Bach Flower Therapy close to a Tarot reading. It is not very beneficial to the credentials of a treatment, if it is (unwillingly) associated with an occult image.

8
THE PRACTICE OF
BACH FLOWER THERAPY

EVALUATION AND CLASSIFICATION USING THE TRACKS
∾

The easiest and most comprehensive way to evaluate a patient is by entering the appropriate flowers into the flow sheet shown in the appendix of this book. It is most practical to use three different colors, representing the following three categories:

1. Flowers that correspond exactly, according to the patient.
2. Flowers that the patient believes are only partially applicable or whose characters are not well defined.
3. Flowers that are seen by the patient as not applicable, but that are viewed by the practitioner as matching ones. Flowers based on organ language belong in this category, as do ones found through astrology. In general, this category embraces flower concepts of which the patient may not be completely aware.

In the following evaluation scheme the flowers of the first category are printed in **bold**, those in the second category in *italics,* and those in the third category in roman.

The interpretation using the tracks should help us first to choose the appropriate flowers for the initial stage of therapy, flowers to treat the more superficial aspects of the problems. If we were to begin with a flower for a more deeply rooted emotional problem, it could lead to unpleasant reactions, especially when the subconscious becomes activated. To avoid this it is recommended that one follow the following hierarchy, which makes the selection of the flowers easier, especially when many flowers are needed.

First Mixture

In principle, the first mixture should contain the following flowers:

1. Star of Bethlehem. Each of us has experienced at some time in our lives an emotional shock. For many people birth already was a shock, especially the moment when they were cut from the umbilical cord, before they started breathing on their own and consequently first experienced the fear of death. Star of Bethlehem therefore belongs in every first bottle, to break down possible existing barriers in the first run. This flower belongs to the outer flowers.
2. All remaining outer flowers, even if the qualities they embody are not seen as strongly developed by the patient. As noted at the beginning, it is possible to work through deeper emotional conflicts only when the mind is no longer occupied by the confrontation with outside factors.
3. The discovered decompensation flowers. Because the total number of flowers should not exceed seven, we may have to restrict ourselves to the most important ones.

Several flowers should be given at the beginning. In many cases the maximum of seven flowers is often given to bring those afflicted out of their phase of decompensation and to prepare them for the treatment of their particular problems. In further mixtures the number of flowers is successively reduced.

If it appears that the interview indicates an extremely large number of flowers, this should be seen as a clue for Wild Oat. If the patient cannot decide because of the multitude of possible flowers, only Wild Oat in conjunction with Star of Bethlehem and the required outer flowers should be given, in order to keep the number of applied flowers as small as possible. This should clarify the situation. After four to six weeks of ingestion, the number of appropriate flowers is drastically reduced in the next follow-up session.

Second Mixture

After approximately four weeks we should reevaluate which of the applied flowers are still required. For this we need to talk again with the patient about the symptoms described at the beginning. Reading them to patients in their own original words seems to work the best, because they have an easier time recognizing them again.

After we mark down the results on a second evaluation sheet, a classification for the second mixture becomes apparent. If we compare the result with the first evaluation sheet we can obtain control information on the progress of the treatment.

We often can see an improvement in situations for which we gave no flowers at all. This can be explained by the fact that the ingestion of the outer flowers and the decompensation flowers means a tremendous relief for the individual. The mind is now able to deal with inner conflicts and situations that were previously blocked as a result of too much suffering. For this reason all flowers determined by the first interview should be reevaluated, not only the ones that have been taken so far. The new mixture is based on the momentary state. In place of the flowers that are no longer needed, we now prescribe flowers determined by the new evaluation. More tracks are often indicated. One should focus on the main problem first, however, and on the flowers needed for it. Both can be recognized according to the following criteria:

1. The intensity of a track can be seen by how deep the individual finds himself in the state of decompensation.
2. In conversation with the patient these flowers are pointed out as the most applicable ones. This is the place of greatest despair.
3. Physical symptoms point to the most intense emotional problems.
4. The most disturbed skin zones in the Bach Flower body maps also reveal the most urgently needed flowers.

One should work from top to bottom that is, on one, two, or at most three tracks; start first of all with the decompensation remedy, followed by the compensation remedy, and finish with the communication remedy.

If only a few flowers are needed or one track is very acute, two flowers from one track can also be given simultaneously, according to the preexisting sequence.

If only the communication flower from one track is indicated, it is possible to add it to the other ones if the flower concept is very distinct. One does not always have to treat from top to bottom. It is possible to give communication flowers before all the compensation states have been cleared up. *All* the decompensation flowers should already have been given, however, before one starts to address deeper states.

If Larch is indicated, it can be given in the second mixture. Most often, however, it will be used in a later state, because as the foundation flower it represents the actual background for the problems and therefore must step back for more acute flowers.

Further Course of Treatment

The respective flower combinations should be evaluated and rearranged in four- to six-week intervals as described above. Once the superficial problems have subsided and the composition of the mixtures no longer changes, it is possible to increase the intervals.

The more deeply situated problems need a much longer application of the flowers, as in the case of more acute problems. In chronic problems it often takes between one and one and a half years to completely resolve them.

After approximately three months some therapists discontinue treatment for two to four weeks to allow the previous remedies to come to their full effect and to see whether an improvement already has been established. The time period without treatment also indicates how well the individuals will be able to get along without the remedies. In this time period they often become more conscious of the flowers they still need.

A pause in the treatment makes sense to clarify the situation, especially if the patient needs many different flowers or has tried many diverse flowers without success. Otherwise, I do not think that it is really necessary.

Case Studies

Example 1. This example demonstrates the method in a simple case. The flowers usually do not fit together as nicely as they do here, and one has to work harder to distinguish clearly which flowers fit the present problem, which apply to situations in the past, and which have only a momentary relevance.

Let us assume that the evaluation gives us the following flowers (the order corresponds to the form of the evaluation sheet used in the appendix):

Pine	Wild Rose	Impatiens
Holly	*Willow*	
Centaury	Gentian	
Larch		
Walnut		*Gorse*

Feelings of guilt are listed as the main problem, along with a lack of assertiveness and the feeling of resignation in situations in which the individual cannot assert himself. Because he feels unfairly treated by his co-workers, he wants to change his career. He even has a new job already lined up; he lacks the courage to make the initial move, however, although his inner impatience is urging him to do so. First mixture: *Star of Bethlehem, Walnut, Gorse, Pine, Wild Rose.*

After the next visit the following situation has evolved: The Wild Rose state has not appeared again. The Walnut symptoms have improved overall but still continue in a mild form. His guilt feelings have not changed much; they seem to be deeply rooted. Second mixture: *Walnut, Pine, Holly, Willow, Impatiens.*

Four weeks later, at the follow-up visit, the following has presumingly happened: The impatience has improved only to a minimal extent. The guilt feelings, however, have ceased altogether. Third mixture: *Holly, Centaury, Impatiens, Larch, Gentian.*

Eight weeks later the clinical picture could look like this: The patient has finally changed his job and despite his low expectations gets along very well. Meanwhile he understands (because of the application of Gentian) that he did not view everything as optimistically as he thought he had. He also does not get angry as easily anymore. His inability to say no is still a problem for him. His self-esteem could also be better, but in the meantime his impatience has disappeared. Fourth mixture: *Centaury, Gentian, Larch.*

The fourth mixture now can be given over a longer period without much control, because it covers the patient's most deeply situated emotional conflicts. In other words, it is his own emotional "constitutional remedy."

Example 2. The symptoms have been left out of the following example because I want only to demonstrate the composition of the flower remedies through the eva-luation of the tracks.

The following result was obtained by the interview:

Pine	Wild Oat	**Wild Rose**	
Holly	*Vine*	*Willow*	
	Cerato	**Gentian**	Clematis
Crab Apple	White Chestnut	Beech	
	Hornbeam	*Chestnut Bud*	
Scleranthus	**Vervain**		
Larch			
Star of Bethlehem		*Gorse*	

The following flowers were prescribed: *Star of Bethlehem, Gorse, Pine, Wild Oat, Wild Rose, Crab Apple, Chestnut Bud.* Using the Bach Flower body maps, *Pine, Wild Rose,* and *Star of Bethlehem* were applied externally in the form of compresses. The flower remedies were taken for three-and-a-half months in this combination with periodic control visits. Subsequently, the following clinical picture evolved:

Pine Holly	Vine	*Wild Rose* Willow **Gentian**
	White Chestnut **Hornbeam** **Vervain**	Beech *Chestnut Bud*
Star of Bethlehem	**Elm**	

The condition significantly improved overall. The feeling of desperation (Gorse) completely disappeared. Instead, an acute Elm state originated because of the external situation.

It was apparent that the Holly and the Vine states improved, although these flowers themselves had not been given; only the corresponding decompensation flowers were given. This phenomenon can be seen quite frequently and shows us the composition of the flowers within the track. The other flower states within the track will often respond if relief is achieved through the application of one flower.

The subsequent mixture was composed of the following: *Star of Bethlehem, Elm, Willow, Wild Rose, Hornbeam, Vervain, Chestnut Bud.* White Chestnut and Beech were not used because they existed only in a latent state and did not present a problem at the moment. The most urgently needed flowers were Hornbeam and Vervain.

During the further course of treatment only *Gentian* would be added, provided that no other external circumstances created the need for more flowers. Otherwise, the unnecessary flowers would be left out and the number of flowers thereby reduced.

Example 3. In this example the astrological signs are also given because they show an interesting correspondence. Some flowers that were not obvious in the horoscope were also chosen. The negative emotional states of the Centaury state were listed as the main problem:

Vervain **Agrimony** Sun and Mercury	**Pine** **Holly** **Centaury** Saturn	Cerato	**Chicory** Ruler of the Ascendant and Moon
Willow Gentian	**Olive**	**Scleranthus** Ascendant	Beech **Chestnut Bud**
Larch			
Star of Bethlehem		Gorse	

As confusing as this picture looks at first glimpse—after all, sixteen flowers are applicable—the hierarchical classification is easy with the help of the tracks. The sequence of mixtures is:

1. All necessary outer flowers: *Star of Bethlehem, Gorse*
2. All necessary decompensation flowers, as long the total number of applied flowers does not exceed seven: *Pine, Beech.*
3. Compensation flowers in the sequence the patient believes they are necessary: *Holly, Olive, Willow.*

The foundation flower, *Larch,* can be added to the remaining flowers in the second mixture.

Example 4. The last example again portrays a case in which seventeen flowers—almost every other one—could be used. Interpretation using the tracks helps in such an extreme case to bring order to this chaos and to provide the therapy with a clear line.

The interview produced the following flowers:

Pine	**Wild Oat**	Cherry Plum
Holly		**Agrimony**
Centaury	Cerato	
Wild Rose	White Chestnut	Mustard
Willow	Hornbeam	**Impatiens**
Gentian	*Vervain*	
Star of Bethlehem		*Walnut*

The main problem is characterized through the Centaury track. This was also the position of the moon in the astrological interpretation. The following mixture was prescribed: *Star of Bethlehem, Pine, Wild Oat, Wild Rose, Cherry Plum, Mustard.*

Three months later the following picture evolved:

Pine	Wild Oat	Agrimony
Holly		
Centaury	Cerato	
Wild Rose		Impatiens
Gentian	*Vervain*	
Star of Bethlehem		**Walnut**

As in the second example, the deeper states also improved in this case through the application of the decompensation flowers.

The worsening of the Walnut state can be explained by the fact that the flower was not given, although it represents an external flower and actually should have been given priority. Through the ingestion of the flowers something starts to move on the psychological level, and the superficial symptoms are more noticeable if they are not treated. The Holly state has been intensified by the prescription of Pine. This can be explained by a decrease in feelings of guilt, which causes the patient to feel less timid.

This phenomenon can often be observed and indicates that Holly should now be given.

As the second mixture the following flower remedies were prescribed: *Star of Bethlehem, Wild Rose, Holly.* Two months after the start of the new flower combination, only the flower concepts of Holly and Star of Bethlehem were still strong, whereas Vervain was now evaluated as medium strong. The other states had either subsided or existed in a subliminal form. This case shows us that a consequent use of the tracks will systematically reduce the number of flowers until at the very end only a few flowers remain, which represent the emotional "constitutional remedy." This one should be given over a long time period.

One should not be confused by examples in the literature with one to three flowers. In those cases probably only the most pronounced symptoms were treated. It also could have been the case that those examples were chosen to explain the clinical picture of one flower.

A detailed interview, however, ususaly yields eight to twelve flowers. The last two case studies were extreme examples, which should demonstrate how the consequent application of the track can relatively easily solve "difficult cases." For all the suitable flowers one should always asks the question, Why does the patient need just this particular flower? Perhaps it treats only the superficial side of a problem, while the actual cause lies hidden at a much deeper level. Bach Flower Therapy calls for a complete work-up and treatment of the problem at hand—that is, if one takes its goal of connecting us again with our higher self.

PREPARATION AND DOSAGES OF THE FLOWER REMEDIES
∾

Preparations for Chronic Ailments

From a stock bottle, place three drops of each flower essence—with Rescue Remedy, six drops—in a one-ounce medicine bottle. (A total number of seven flowers should not be exceeded.) Add a small amount of alcohol (schnapps, brandy, or medical alcohol) for preservation and fill the bottle with uncarbonated mineral water. Water with a high calcium content can cause precipitation; therefore, watch the mineral content. The ratio between water and alcohol should be approximately three to one. With high-proof alcohol, use less.

For children one can reduce the alcohol content by frequently preparing fresh mixtures. For alcoholics one should leave out the alcohol additive completely in favor of a mixture with a much shorter shelf life.

As with all the naturopathic medicines the Bach Flower Remedies should under no circumstances be refrigerated. Direct sunlight and strong electro-magnetic fields should be avoided as well. The flowers should not be placed on the TV or on speakers.

One should take two to four drops four times a day from the solution. The first ingestion should happen preferably in the morning on an empty stomach, the second just before lunch, the third just before dinner, and the last before going to bed. If necessary, one can also take a higher dose and take the flowers more frequently without any trouble. Edward Bach himself wrote that dosage does not matter so much, because none of the remedies can cause the smallest amount of damage, even if taken in large amounts—although a small dosage is sufficient.[1]

Many patients develop a feeling over time for how many drops they need. Sometimes these people also feel when the time has come to change the mixture, by developing an instinctive aversion to the ingestion of the flowers. In sensitive patients it is possible to reduce the dosage when strong reactions occur. One can also dilute the drops in a glass of water and let the patient sip it one or two times a day.

Preparations for Acute Ailments

In acute cases, add two drops (with Rescue Remedy four drops) from the stock bottle to one glass of water, from which the patient should drink one sip every fifteen to thirty minutes—in extreme cases, even every five minutes. In emergency situations Rescue Remedy can be given directly from the stock bottle onto the tongue. In my practice I give it immediately after a circulatory preparation in case of a collapse, because it will quickly take away the fear that often occurs in those situations.

The outer flowers are also suitable for such a dilution in water. Elm, for example, taken in small sips of water before tests or games, prevents black-outs, if necessary in conjunction with Rescue Remedy and Olive. In cases of low self-esteem one should give Larch, along with with other suitable flow-ers, in normal preparation over a long time period. Because problems with self-esteem are usually deeply rooted, a short treatment is usually insufficient. Rescue Remedy and Olive, however, are only taken *prior* to a game.

For the immediate care after an emotional shock or disappointment, Star of Bethlehem is also better used in diluted form than in the normal prepara-tion. One usually gives Rescue Remedy in those cases, however, because it also contains other emergency flowers, such as Rock Rose, for panic.

Walnut diluted in water also helps much faster in situations in which time is especially critical. Some practitioners divide up the diagnosed flowers into chronic and acute ones and always give the latter in the form of water dilution.

Other Forms of Application

External application in the form of compresses and ointments. Bach Flower Remedies can also be applied topically. For the compresses, add two drops of each flower essence into one-quarter cup of water and wet a cloth with it. This mixture should always be freshly prepared for each application. It is also advisable to use disposable cloths, because eczema and open wounds could spread germs onto the cloth and in any case transfers imbalanced energetic information.

For the ointment add two drops of each flower essence to 10g of a salve base, which can be a neutral ointment base or an already prepared cream. Adding essential oils or other ingredients does not influence the effect. The flower remedy should be well dispersed by stirring it into the ointment for a long time. Rescue Remedy is already available as an ointment. In case of burns one can apply Rescue Remedy in pure form or as an ointment on the skin. In this way, the development of blisters can be stopped in many cases, and the healing can be increased.

For rashes the following flowers should be considered:

> Crab Apple: for cleansing
> Holly: for infection or itching
> Cherry Plum: to fight the urge to scratch
> Pine: for possible feelings of guilt if the patient scratches the sores
>   open and bloody

Pine is also the decompensation flower of Holly. The other flowers are all decompensation flowers. For extreme physical reactions—for example, rashes and allergies—decompensation flowers and outer flowers (mainly Star of Bethlehem) are usually needed.

Bach Flower/Baths. A few drops from the stock bottle may be added to the bath water. The flower Olive creates a popular regeneration bath. In states of exhaustion caused by mental overload, use a Hornbeam bath. As an addition to the flowers given orally, we can add some drops of Crab Apple into the bath water for rashes.

Additives to baths do not interfere with the effect of the flowers.

Eye drops. Bach Flower Remedies may also be applied in form of eye drops. For these we must keep some things in mind to prevent an eye infection.

Only sterile eye droppers should be used; they can be bought in every pharmacy. As a base solution one should use normal isotonic saline solution, preferably in small vials for injection purposes. The mixing should be done with disposable syringes. Under no circumstances can alcohol be used, because it irritates the eyes. We must also use extreme caution so that the dropper does not touch the eye. The solution lasts as long it is not contaminated by an external source. Two drops of each flower essence should be added. Star of Bethlehem has proven especially beneficial for eye injuries and conjunctivitis.

Some practitioners also apply eye drops for far- and near-sightedness. I did not find any results, but success is possible. An American physician, Dr. Bates, was able to show that not only the pupil but the whole eye is capable of adapting and glasses can often be discarded after long-term eye training. (See Harry Benjamin, *Better Sight Without Glasses* [San Francisco: Thorsons, 1986].)

Nasal spray. The flowers can also be applied as a nasal spray. Again, no alcohol can be used, because it would irritate the mucus membranes inside the nose. As with the eye drops, an isotonic saline solution is recommended, but it is also possible to add the drops to ready-made (if possible natural) nose drops.

For the common cold, the following flowers should be considered:

Crab Apple: for cleansing
Holly: for irritation of the mucus membranes
Star of Bethlehem: in cases of trauma, for example, cold air, draft, chills
Olive: for immune deficiency caused by overwork
Pine: for feelings of guilt, because other people feel disturbed by the constant sneezing and nose blowing

In cases of hay fever we should also consider the following flowers:

Beech: as a result of allergies
Cherry Plum: to fight the urge to sneeze

I must emphasize again that the Bach Flower Remedies should not be prescribed based on the symptoms of an illness. Although the suggested flowers originate through the organ language, their use should always be discussed with the patient and applied on an individual basis. For example, a trivial cold can hide a deeply rooted inner conflict—the individual might be chronically "stuffed up," maybe even embittered. The physical symptoms are the attempt of the body to bring a suppressed emotional conflict to the surface with the help of the organ language.

Take-along bottles. Some practitioners let their patients carry the flower mixture in small bottles on the body to intensify their effect. It is also possible to tape the individual flowers in small containers on the corresponding skin areas to achieve a long-lasting effect in therapy-resistant problems.

To place a bottle containing the flowers under the pillow at night is also a popular form of application. The patient often reports increased dream activity.

The different flower application methods seem to have no set limits, and one can use one's imagination. Ear irrigation might work in corresponding problems, as might hair tinctures when one wants to tear out one's hair in anger, or even enemas for diarrhea or the cleaning of the colon.

One method of application, however, has not been shown to be beneficial after all: the injection. Because the flowers are based on energetic information, it does not matter whether they are applied on or under the skin. Ointment rubbed onto the corresponding area of the skin has proven to be the most effective in comparison with other methods of application.

Reaction to the Ingestion

Some people experience an instant sensation of relief after the ingestion. This is especially the case in very sensitive people. For them an improvement often happens very quickly.

In general, however, it will be very slow in the first weeks but then will continuously improve. Although the actual ailments do not get better immediately, improvement in the overall constitution is noted, along with the feeling that something is happening. A positive attitude toward the seemingly insurmountable problems can often be felt.

In some cases a *primary aggravation* may occur. Physical as well as emotional complaints can increase. Under certain circumstances the individual may suffer under extreme mood swings. If the flowers are discontinued, these unpleasant appearances quickly fade away; one thus need not fear these primary aggravations. The reaction shows after all that something is moving psychologically and therefore should be seen in a positive light.

After the state is somewhat diminished, the flowers should be given again in a lower dosage. The number of drops should be chosen such that no further reaction will appear. If necessary the drops should be diluted in a glass of water, and the patient should drink one sip once or twice a day. Some brave people continue to take the drops at the same dosage and consciously withstand the unpleasant reaction in order to gain some insight into themselves. Repressed feelings often reemerge and the individuals recognize what has made them "sick."

If the unpleasant reactions reoccur despite a reduction in the dosage, one should examine whether an important flower is missing from the mixture. I have often been able to observe how the ingestion of Centaury magnified existing guilt feelings. This makes sense because the offering of a communication flower will push a patient even further into decompensation. If we work with the tracks we can avoid those situations completely. Since I started working with this method, primary aggravations have occurred very rarely.

Working with flower combinations based exclusively on the astrological method produces a much higher number of primary aggravation states, and in some cases even relatively dramatic psychological reactions.

Dreams

Dreams come from the subconscious mind. They can show symbolically how Bach Flower Therapy works in this space that is inaccessible to the waking mind. There is usually an increase in dream activity anyway, and many patients tell about their dreams on their own. Because indicative dreams may occur as early as the first night following the first ingestion of the flowers, one should make the patient aware of them and ask her to write them down. These dreams often indicate which problem is being worked on at the moment. It does not require an elaborate knowledge of dream interpretation to determine whether the flowers are suitable or not.

A dream that is perceived as clearly unpleasant or even threatening and is recurring can indicate a problem that has not been addressed by the flower combination. The dream is often so obvious in its meaning that the individual herself recognizes the particular problem, and the search for the appropriate flower should then be no problem.

If a person appears in these dreams to scold the dreamer, it can be referred to Pine (criticism produces guilt feelings) or to Larch (as a result of embarrassment).

Haunting dreams indicate that the individual is running away from something in her life. A talk can clarify the particular cause. If the individual constantly runs away from unpleasant situations, it could be interpreted as pointing to Chestnut Bud.

Terrifying dreams symbolize subconscious elements that are seen as threatening. Cherry Plum would be the appropriate flower for this state, but one should also consider Rock Rose (for panic) and Aspen (for eerie feelings of fear). If terrifying dreams occur *as a result* of the flower treatment, however, only Cherry Plum should be considered.

Barriers

Treatment sometimes fails, although the flowers were chosen in the right way. In her article published in the *Bach Newsletter,* J. Evans offers the following reasons:

1. Illness as a chance to learn
2. The wrong moment
3. The patient wants to hold on to his illness
4. Willful rejection
5. Lack of persistence

Response to 1. An illness sometimes represents an attempt by the body to force the patient to change her life circumstances. If she continues to make the same mistakes, however—if she works too much, or goes to bed too late, or gets up too early and drinks too much coffee to prop herself up—then healing is not possible.

Response to 2. The patient has still not learned the whole lesson of her illness. For example, she may not drink coffee anymore, but continues to go to bed late. Her complaints of fatigue, headaches, and inner states of tension that are caused by lack of sleep will only vanish if she gives her body the needed rest. In this regard the flower Olive, for example, can be misused to exploit the body even further.

Response to 3. There are people who constantly need therapists for their inner dissatisfaction or boredom. After the existing complaints have faded away, they produce new symptoms according to their needs. These complaints are usually relatively vague: sometimes it hurts in one spot, sometimes in another, and often the individuals suffer from minor complaints.

These patients often turn into nightmares for therapists because real progress in their treatment cannot be seen at all. It is like cutting off the heads of Hydra, and one always has the feeling that the patient does not really care about healing his "pain" but rather enjoys the attention attainable only in treatment. The flower Heather is the only remedy that might produce success, assuming the patient is willing to take it.

Patients sometimes do not want to get better at all. Under certain circumstances they might not even come out of their own free will but rather are pushed into treatment by family members. In these cases the treatment serves only as an alibi for the relatives.

Keep in mind that every illness produces advantages of some kind. For example, one does not need to work, meals are served in bed, and suddenly the relatives have time again for the sick person, which previously was not the case. One has time again for oneself and can read a book that had to be put away for other, more important things. When one thinks twice about it, it is not bad to pay with a little pain and discomfort. For every illness the possibility exists of striking the balance between advantages and disadvantages. According to what predominates, the chances of getting better can quickly be estimated.

Response to 4. Individuals just do not want to believe that these delicate remedies can help. In these cases the subconscious fights the vibration of the flowers, and healing is not possible.

Response to 5. Almost every patient has her favorite symptom, and if this does not vanish immediately, the treatment is judged a failure. For this reason one should always ask in the follow-up visits about all the symptoms found in the first interview. A noticeable improvement can often be seen four to six weeks after the beginning of the flower treatment, so we can assume that the treatment has started to work.

In chronic problems that have existed for years or in emotional problems, patience is required. In naturopathic medicine the rule of thumb is that each illness takes the same number of months to disappear as the number of years it has existed.

Otherwise Bach Flower Therapy offers a treatment for especially rushed patients: "impatience drops" (Impatiens)!

Difficulties with the Patient's Relationships with Others

During treatment problems sometimes arise with the patient's relationships, because these are affected by the flowers no less than the patient's behavior. A Centaury-Vine relationship, for example, will no longer be able to function in the same way, if the weaker one takes Centaury. The Vine partner has to adjust to the new situation, in which he cannot continue his power game. The Centaury partner is now showing more strength, will defend herself against external influences, and will resist playing the emotional trashcan for her partner.

At first the partner interprets this negatively. The patients often complain in the following way: "My spouse tells me that I've changed in a negative way through Bach Flower Therapy. Although I know that I'm on the right track and I don't have to be exploited by others, I still feel insecure."

The so-called negative change expresses itself in a way that the husband has to clean his own shoes now, does not get his bottle of beer served anymore and has to give up the pleasant things in life, which had so far been at the other's expense.

It is important not to leave the patients alone with their flower remedies but to offer them advice, especially with confrontation in the workplace. Here one has to be especially careful, because the colleagues or the boss usually do not have an understanding for the sudden "escapades" of their once goodnatured and helpful co-worker. If they cannot take advantage of her anymore, they have to find some other "naive" person.

One should therefore never forget that others are usually not aware of their egocentric behavior. The situation might have evolved this way over time, and the Centaury colleague has created this behavior through her own excessive helpfulness. Because until now she always voluntarily worked overtime, more and more tasks have gradually fallen to her.

One can imagine how upset her co-workers must be about her changed behavior, especially when she suddenly becomes aware of how much she has been taken advantage of and therefore changes her behavior from one day to the next. I myself have experienced cases in which a whole family or the whole office was turned upside down in no time. One practitioner told me about the son of a patient who moved out of his parents' house because he could not stand the new willpower of his father, who had been taking Centaury for a few weeks.

The Centaury track seems to play an important role, especially in the confrontation with family, friends, and co-workers. According to a statistic I ob-tained in my own practice, Centaury and Pine are the most frequently used flowers.

SELF TREATMENT: POSSIBILITIES AND LIMITS

The simplicity and harmlessness of Bach Flower Therapy make it ideal for the self-treatment of minor ailments and discomforts, and for the general prevention of illness. Applications include:

- Test anxiety
- Travel sickness
- First day of school
- New job
- Effects of overwork
- Tiredness and tension after night work
- Aftereffects of anger
- Results of emotional trauma and shock

∾ Feelings of guilt after failure
∾ All the indications for Rescue Remedy (see below)
∾ Treatment of animals and plants

Proven flower combinations

TEST DROPS (ACCORDING TO JULIAN BARNARD)[2]

Gentian:	for doubts and discouragement
Elm:	for the temporary loss of self-esteem
Clematis:	for the dream-like, absentminded state
Larch:	for feelings of inadequacy or failure
White Chestnut:	to enhance concentration

COMBINATION FOR THE FIRST DAY OF SCHOOL[3]

Honeysuckle:	for homesickness
Mimulus:	for insecurity and fear of new situations
Walnut:	for the change into a new phase in life
Olive:	for exhaustion that results from expending psychological energy in new situations

---

COMBINATION FOR TRAVEL SICKNESS
(SEASICKNESS OR FEAR AND DIZZINESS IN AIRPLANES)[4]

Scleranthus:	for vertigo
Rescue Remedy:	for general excitement

COMBINATION TO HELP ONE STOP SMOKING
(ACUPUNCTURE CAN ALSO BE BENEFICIAL)

Agrimony:	for addiction
Cherry Plum:	for compulsive behavior (especially in chain smokers); for the feeling of going crazy without nicotine
Larch:	to build up self-esteem
Centaury:	for a lack of willpower
Gentian:	for doubts about success
Walnut:	to facilitate physiological and psychological change

Indications for Rescue Remedy

- Injuries
- Burns (applied externally)
- Accidents (as a first-aid measure until the physician has arrived)
- Before and after surgery
- Pain
- Fainting
- Delirium (as a first-aid measure until the physician has arrived)
- Dental appointment
- Date of a divorce
- Receiving bad news
- Tragedies
- Conflicts
- Breakdown caused by overwork
- Insomnia caused by stress or when "wound up"
- After a horror movie

If there is no exact diagnosis or one does not know which flower to take, one can always apply the rule of thumb for self-treatment: "For an emergency, always Rescue Remedy." The situations in which Rescue Remedy is appropriate are those in which self-treatment is most likely to be needed. Gregory Vlamis describes in his book *Bach Flower Remedies to the Rescue* successful treatments with Rescue Remedy in approximately 190 cases.

Prevention of Illness

Edward Bach wrote that just as moods can lead us to the right way of treatment, they can also serve as an early warning for imminent conditions and thereby offer us the opportunity to stop the attack. Prior to almost all physical complaints is a time in which we do not feel completely fit or feel somewhat exhausted. At this time it is necessary to treat our state of being to prevent a more severe outbreak.[5]

Limits of Self-Treatment

Physical symptoms should be examined by the physicians or naturopaths before one starts self-treatment, because a more serious disease can sometimes hide behind harmless symptoms. Pain is an alarm symptom and should be treated only if the cause is known.

In apparent illnesses Bach Flower Therapy can easily be combined with every other form of therapy. The effect of other medications, even of high-potency homeopathic remedies, is not influenced by Bach Flowers, which can speed up the healing process and intensify the effect of other treatment methods. They often work as a catalytic agent.

If the degree of the illness permits it, naturopathic medications are preferable to allopathic ones, because the latter often suppress the symptoms at the physical level. Bach Flower Therapy, on the other hand, tries to work with them at the emotional level.

Serious emotional problems belong in the care of an experienced therapist. I advise strongly against self-treatment in such cases, which require much experience and subtle intuition. Deeply situated emotional problems and inner conflicts cannot be treated on one's own. No one is completely honest with himself, a fact that makes finding the appropriate flowers for deep problems an insurmountable obstacle. Although astrology can provide many useful clues, they must be interpreted objectively and seen in relation to the current situation.

To oversee the effect of the flower combination, to interpret reactions such as primary aggravation, dreams, and so forth, in the right way—this exceeds the capabilities of the individual. As already mentioned, family, friends, and co-workers will react to the patient's altered behavior; thus a counterpart is necessary, someone who can evaluate the whole problem in an objective way.

From experience we know that people who find their flower combination with the help of a therapist are later able to treat themselves on their own with Bach Flowers. For example, they are able to cure themselves of respiratory infections, colds, coughs, and so on, by means of Bach Flowers. This is possible because in the meantime they have experienced their strong and weak sides and therefore are now able to recognize their flaws in acute problems.

The goal of a treatment should be to release the patient at a later point into self-sufficiency. The task of practitioners is, as an old naturopathic idiom says, to make themselves obsolete.

Treatment of Animals

Animals respond extremely well to Bach Flower Therapy. Because animals cannot communicate with words, one must rely entirely on observation, which requires sensitivity and diagnostic ability.

If, for example, a dog has acted crazy since his owner got a second dog, jealousy is the likely cause. In this case we should consider Holly. If he has stopped eating since he was clawed by the neighbor's cat, one should use Star of Bethlehem to help him overcome the shock. If he tucks his tail between his legs even when he sees much smaller dogs, Larch can strengthen his self-esteem.

A parrot always retreated, loudly shrieking, into the furthest corner of his cage as soon someone approached him. After several doses of Rock Rose he lost his panicky fear and was actually able to approach people.

One practitioner told me: "I treated a patient over a long period of time, and every time I saw her in the office I noticed that the backs of her hands were covered with scratches. When I asked her what had happened to her hands, she replied that her tomcat Felix would always scratch and bite her. This would happen only when she pet the other cat first and touched Felix afterward. After the situation had quieted down, he would be the most cuddly cat again, and she never could be angry at him."

Felix was obviously jealous when he was not petted first. He reacted aggressively and scratched his owner's hand. Later on he obviously developed guilt feelings and wanted to make up by acting gentle.

The patient was advised to add Holly and Pine to his daily milk. After one week she happily came back and reported that Felix had completely changed. The treatment had already been successful on the second day. She proudly showed her hands to me and said: "The tomcat doesn't act aggressive anymore. On the contrary, he no longer needs any caressing from me because he receives it now from the other cat, to whom he attends in a caring way."

As the treatment of animals requires some experience in Bach Flower Therapy, I suggest Rescue Remedy drops for first trials. Most of the acute problems occur as a result of external influences, so emergency drops as a universal remedy rarely fail to have an effect.

"Character flaws" in animals are somewhat harder to cure. Perhaps the now more trendy animal astrology will offer some diagnostic clues. Very interesting is the fact that animals often need the same flowers as their owners. As animals often imitate the behavior of people, they also seem to take over their attitudes.

Treatment of Houseplants

Houseplants also respond very well to Bach Flower Therapy. Two drops of a flower may be added to the water directly from the stock bottle.

The well-known Backster experiments in the 1960s established that plants do indeed have feelings. Because plants communicate even less than animals, one must rely completely on assumptions. Only dropped flowers and brown or dropped leaves indicate that something is missing for the plant.

If these problems occur after repotting, one can give Walnut as the flower for a new beginning or Star of Bethlehem for shock.

If the plant was also relocated, one could also consider Walnut, if it does not get along in its new surroundings, Honeysuckle also could be considered for possible homesickness.

Some plants feel offended after repotting, if they are no longer the center of attention and therefore receive less affection. In those cases Heather is the flower of choice.

If problems start to occur after one forgets to water the plant, one should think of Star of Bethlehem, the flower for shock, or Rock Rose, for the potential fear of death. If the plant does not recuperate, Wild Rose should be chosen for resignation.

Crab Apple should be very helpful against bugs of all kinds.

Case Studies

A schefflera plant dropped its leaves after it had to move from its place at the balcony door to a new place close to a big window. At the same time, another houseplant at the windowsill dropped its leaves. Both plants were in a desolate state; my wife had already given up on them. The schefflera received Holly, because it obviously envied the other plant its place at the windowsill. The other plant received Heather, because it was obviously hurt by the schefflera aggression and probably dropped its leaves out of plain self-pity. Both plants recuperated within days.

A colleague wrote to me about two other examples:

When I opened up my office I received a palm tree as a present that looked strong and healthy. After a while, however, the palm tree started to become pale and wilted. It looked as if the leaves were turning gray and brown from the outside going in.

I asked for advice at a floral shop, to see whether I had done something wrong that might have harmed the plant. This, however, was negated. I decided to add three drops of Walnut to the tree's water to help it get used to the new environment. The palm tree became better in a few days and now looks as beautiful as it did the first day.

In a beauty parlor stood a beautiful Jojoba palm tree that everyone admired. When another plant was placed right in front of it, however, and the palm tree was less visible at first glance, many leaves suddenly started to wither. After it was brought back to the front, it recuperated again. As an experiment it was placed again behind the other flower, but this time Heather and Holly were added to the water. No negative reaction occurred this time, and even today it is as beautiful as ever, although it has taken the place in the back.

As a more detailed differentiation of the flower remedies requires more experience in the handling of Bach Flowers and also some intuition, I recommend for the first trials, just as in the treatment of animals, the use of Rescue Remedy.

Appendix

Questionnaire
∾

1. *Are there situations in which you are afraid?*
    (Aspen, Mimulus, Rock Rose, Cherry Plum, Red Chestnut, Larch, Centaury, Crab Apple)

2. *Are there situations in which you feel insecure?*
    (Cerato, Scleranthus, Wild Oat, Gentian, Hornbeam)

3. *Do you sometimes lack concentration? Are you easily distracted from your work?*
    (Clematis, Honeysuckle, White Chestnut, Chestnut Bud, Wild Rose, Mustard, Olive)

4. *Do you sometimes feel lonely?*
    (Heather, Water Violet, Impatiens)

5. *In what situations are you influenced by others?*
    (Centaury, Walnut, Holly, Agrimony)

6. *Are there situations in which you feel discouraged or desperate?*
    (Star of Bethlehem, Sweet Chestnut, Willow, Crab Apple, Pine, Larch, Elm, Oak)

7. *Do you worry about the well-being of other people?*
    (Chicory, Vine, Beech, Vervain, Rock Water)

8. *To what do you react sensitively?*
    (Mimulus, Agrimony, Larch, Pine, Vervain, Impatiens, Centaury, Gentian, Chicory)

9. *What do you think about when you have time to think?*
    (Star of Bethlehem, Honeysuckle, Clematis, White Chestnut, Willow, Chestnut Bud, Red Chestnut)

10. *What makes you angry?*
    (Holly, Centaury, Vervain, Rock Water, Beech, Impatiens)

11. *What is dissatisfying to you at the moment?*
    (Chicory, Wild Oat, Vervain, Pine, Rock Water, Impatiens, Hornbeam, Water Violet)

12. *What makes you feel exhausted?*
    (Olive, Hornbeam, Elm, Oak, Centaury)

13. *What keeps you from being completely happy?*
    (Holly, Wild Oat, Wild Rose, Gorse, Sweet Chestnut, Pine, Crab Apple, Rock Water, Vervain, Star of Bethlehem, Scleranthus, Gentian, Mustard, Water Violet, Agrimony, Hornbeam, Olive)

14. *Do you sometimes feel sad and blue?*
    (Mustard, Gentian, Wild Oat, Gorse, Sweet Chestnut)

15. *Are you careless about minor details or are you a perfectionist?*

    ### Careless, sloppy:
    (Wild Rose, Wild Oat, Clematis, Chestnut Bud, Water Violet, Heather, Hornbeam, Mustard)

    ### Perfectionist:
    (Crab Apple, Vervain, Rock Water, Water Violet, Heather, Centaury)

16. *Do you mind if you have to wait?*
    (Impatiens, Cherry Plum, Holly, Beech, Gentian)

17. *Do you frequently make the same mistakes?*
    (Chestnut Bud, Clematis, Centaury)

18. *Do you sometimes have the feeling that you are superior to other people?*
    (Water Violet, Rock Water)

19. *Do you tend to have feelings of guilt?*
    (Pine, Crab Apple)

20. *Do you feel jealousy and envy?*
    (Holly)

21. *Do you feel you have been unfairly treated by someone? Is there someone whom you cannot forgive? Do you know the feeling of bitterness?*
    (Willow)

22. *Do you sometimes feel unclean in some way? Are you bothered by dirt? Are you disgusted by other people's toilets? Do you feel disgusted by spiders and snakes?*
(Crab Apple)

23. *Is it sometimes hard for you to make a decision? How do you behave when you have to make a decision?*
(Cerato, Scleranthus, Wild Oat, Walnut, Hornbeam)

24. *Are you more of an optimist or a pessimist?*
(Gentian, Agrimony)

25. *Do you sometimes wish you had more self-esteem? Can you speak in public?*
(Larch, Cerato, Centaury)

26. *How do assert yourself in your environment? What do you do when other people have a completely different opinion from yours? What would you do if you had to do something that you resent with all your heart?*
(Vervain, Vine, Chicory, Impatiens, Rock Water)

27. *How do you react to unpleasant things?*

Anger:
(Holly, Centaury, Water Violet, Beech, Larch)

Sorrow:
(Heather, Star of Bethlehem, Agrimony, Gentian, Gorse)

28. *Do you like to be comforted when you are sad?*
(Agrimony, Heather)

29. *Do you solve your problems on your own or with the help of others?*

Alone:
(Agrimony, Water Violet)

With others:
(Cerato, Heather)

30. *Are there things you consciously avoid because they go against your principles?*
(Rock Water)

31. *Are you a good listener, or do you sometimes take over a conversation?*
(Vervain, Heather, Impatiens)

32. *What do you worry about?*
(Heather, Red Chestnut, Chicory, Gentian)

33. *Have you ever been without hope, resigned? Did you ever give up in your life?*
(Gentian, Gorse, Sweet Chestnut, Wild Rose)

34. *Have you ever had experiences that shocked you?*
(Star of Bethlehem)

35. *Do you have thoughts that you can't let go and that constantly occupy you? Do you talk to yourself sometimes?*
(White Chestnut, Clematis, Pine)

36. *Are there situations that weigh heavily on you? In what kind of situation do you feel tense?*
(Impatiens, Vervain, Agrimony, Oak, Rock Water, Cherry Plum, Beech)

37. *Are there situations in which you react intolerantly?*
(Beech, Rock Water, Vervain, Heather, Holly)

38. *What annoys you the most? What would you most like to change about yourself?*

EVALUATION SHEET

Name: _____

Decompensation flower	Sweet Chestnut	Pine	Wild Oat	Honeysuckle	Mustard	Wild Rose
Compensation flower	Vervain	Holly	Vine	Red Chestnut	Impatiens	Willow
Communication flower	Agrimony	Centaury	Cerato	Chicory	Clematis	Gentian
Zodiac sign	Sagitarius	Virgo	Gemini	Scorpio	Cancer	Taurus

Decompensation flower	Oak	Mustard	Cherry Plum	Crab Apple	White Chestnut	Beech
Compensation flower	Olive	Heather	Agrimony	Rock Water	Hornbeam	Chestnut Bud
Communication flower	Impatiens	Mimulus	Rock Rose	Scleranthus	Vervain	Water Violet
Zodiac sign	Aries	Capricorn	Pisces	Libra	Leo	Aquarius

Foundation flower	Larch

External flower	Aspen	Elm	Gorse	Walnut	Star of Bethlehem

RESOURCES
FOR BACH FLOWER REMEDIES

The original Bach Flower Remedies are still collected today at the same sites used by Edward Bach and prepared according to his method. They are exported by the Dr. Edward Bach Center under the name "Bach Flower Stock Concentrate." These original flower essences can be purchased individually or (for a much better price) as a complete set.

ENGLAND

Bach Flower Remedies Ltd.
Dr. Edward Bach Center
Mount Vernon
Sotwell, Wallingford
Oxfordshire OX10 0PZ
England

NORTH AMERICA

Ellon (Bach USA), Inc.
P.O. Box 320
Woodmere, NY 11598
USA
Tel.: (516) 593-2206

AUSTRALIA

The Parmaceutical Plant Company
P.O. Box 68
Bayswater, Victoria 3153
Australia
Tel.: 03-762 8577/8522

Martin & Pleasance Wholesale Pty Ltd.
P.O. Box 4
Collingwood, Victoria 3066
Australia
Tel.: 419-9733

INDIA

Health Services Society
Krishnamoorty
16/3 Varudhi Nagar
Srirangam, Trichy 620 006
India

Another manufacturer who also prepares flower essences according to Edward Bach's instructions is Healing Herbs (Julian and Martine Barnard). These remedies can be ordered through the following address:

Healing Health Ltd.
P.O. Box 65
GB-Hereford HR2 OUW
England

NOTES

CHAPTER 1. THE BACH FLOWER REMEDIES

1. Edward Bach, "Ye Suffer from Yourselves," in Gregory Vlamis, *Bach Flower Remedies to the Rescue* (Rochester, Vt.: Healing Arts Press, 1990), 120–21.
2. Ibid., 121
3. Ibid.
4. Mechthild Scheffer, *Bach Flower Therapy: Theory and Practice* (Rochester, Vt.: Healing Arts Press, 1988), 16.
5. Ibid., 17.

CHAPTER 3. INNER FLOWERS: THE TWELVE TRACKS

1. Dr. Götz Blome, *Mit Blumen heilen* (Freiburg, Germany: Bauer, 1986), 78.
2. Ibid., 197.
3. Dr. Thomas Verny, *Das Seelenleben des Ungeborenen* (Munich: Rogner and Bernard, 1981), 89.
4. Blome, *Mit Blumen heilen*, 250.
5. Philip Chancellor, *The Handbook of the Bach Flower Remedies* (New Canaan, Conn.: Keats, 1980).
6. Scheffer, *Bach Flower Therapy*, 93.
7. Blome, *Mit Blumen heilen*, 266.

CHAPTER 5. OUTER FLOWERS

1. Verny, *Seelenleben*, 84.
2. Thorwald Dethlefsen, *Schicksal als Chance* (Munich: Goldmann, 1982), 223.

.3. Verny, *Seelenleben,* 16.
4. Blome, *Mit Blumen heilen,* 192.
5. Ibid., 256.

Chapter 6. Rescue Remedy

1. Chancellor, *Handbook.*

Chapter 7. Discovering the Appropriate Flower

1. Blome, *Mit Blumen heilen,* 237.
2. Thorwald Dethlefsen, *Krankheit als Weg* (Munich: Bertlesmann, n.d.), 133.
3. Edward Bach, *Gesammelte Werke* (Grafing: Aquamarin, 1988), 152.
4. Ibid., 47.
5. Ibid., 114.
6. Peter Damian, *The Twelve Healers of the Zodiac: The Astrology Handbook of the Bach Flower Remedies* (York Beach, Me.: Weiser, 1986).
7. Ibid.

Chapter 8. The Practice of Bach Flower Therapy

1. Bach, *Gesammelte Werke,* 88.
2. Julian Barnard, *The Guide to the Bach Flower Remedies* (Saffron Walden, Essex: Daniel, 1979).
3. Ibid.
4. Ibid.
5. Bach, *Gesammelte Werke,* 25–26.

FURTHER READING

The Back Flower Remedies. New Canaan, Conn.: Keats, 1977. Includes *Heal Thyself* and *The Twelve Healers and Other Remedies* by Edward Bach and *The Bach Remedies Repertory* by F. J. Wheeler.

Barnard, Julian. *The Guide to the Bach Flower Remedies.* Saffron Walden, Essex: Daniel, 1971.

Chancellor, Philip. *The Handbook of the Bach Flower Remedies.* New Canaan, Conn.: Keats, 1980.

Damian, Peter. *The Twelve Healers of the Zodiac: The Astrology Handbook of the Bach Flower Remedies.* York Beach, Me.: Weiser, 1986.

Scheffer, Mechthild. *Bach Flower Therapy: Theory and Practice.* Rochester, Vt.: Healing Arts Press, 1988.

Vlamis, Gregory. *Bach Flower Remedies to the Rescue.* Rochester, Vt.: Healing Arts Press, 1990.

Weeks, Nora. *The Medical Discoveries of Edward Bach, Physician.* New Canaan, Conn.: Keats, 1979.

Index

Bach Flower Therapy
Theory and Practice

Mechthild Scheffer

A practitioner and a Bach Centre representative in Germany, Austria, and Switzerland, Scheffer presents a contemporary approach to healing with the Bach Flower Remedies. She describes the flower essences in such a way that you will gain deeper insight into the remedies' underlying psychological concepts, thereby enhancing the potential for self-healing. She includes a comprehensive review of the 38 Bach Flower Remedies and a listing of symptoms for easier diagnosis.
ISBN 0-89281-239-7
$12.95 pb

Bach Flower Remedies
to the Rescue

Gregory Vlamis

Most widely known of all the Bach Flower Remedies is the Rescue Remedy—an emergency first-aid treatment that effectively reduces stress and stabilizes emotional upset during trauma. The author cites several case histories, and includes rare photographs and writings from Dr. Bach's own collection.
"This book and the Bach Flower Rescue Remedy should be in every health care professional's armamentarium, in every home, vehicle, and first aid kit."
—**J. Herbert Fill, M.D.**, psychiatrist and former New York City Commissioner of Mental Health
ISBN 0-89281-378-4
$10.95 pb

AROMATHERAPY: SCENT AND PSYCHE
USING ESSENTIAL OILS FOR PHYSICAL
AND EMOTIONAL WELL-BEING

Peter and Kate Damian

Drawing on the latest research and their professional experience as aromatherapists, the authors examine many applications of aromatic oils, from treating viral infections with garlic or black pepper oil to using rose oil to relax patients undergoing chemotherapy. They detail the use of aromatics from the healing traditions of China, India, Persia, and Egypt, and explain our modern-day scientific understanding of the physiology and psychology of scent. They profile 44 essential oils and provide instruction for creating blends.
ISBN 0-89281-530-2
$16.95 pb

These and other Inner Traditions/Healing Arts Press titles are available at many fine bookstores or, to order directly from the publisher, send a check or money order for the total amount, payable to Inner Traditions, plus $3.00 shipping and handling for the first book and $1.00 for each additional book to:

Inner Traditions
P.O. Box 388
Rochester, VT 05767

Be sure to request a free catalog.